THE PASSIONATE NONSMOKER'S BILL OF RIGHTS

THE PASSIONATE NONSMOKER'S BILL OF RIGHTS

The First Guide to Enacting Nonsmoking Legislation

Steve Allen and Bill Adler, Jr.

William Morrow and Company, Inc. New York

Copyright © 1989 by Bill Adler Books, Inc.

Grateful acknowledgment is made for permission to use the following:

Environmental Tobacco Smoke: Measuring Exposures and Assessing Health Effects.
Copyright © 1986 by the National Academy of Sciences, Washington, D.C.

O'Hara, John H. "Radioactivity and Cigarette Smoke" [letter]. *New York State Journal of Medicine,* December 1983. Reprinted by permission from the *New York State Journal of Medicine,* copyright © 1983 by the Medical Society of the State of New York.

Smith, David. "Absenteeism and Presenteeism in Industry." *Archives of Environmental Health,* November 1970. Reprinted with permission of the Helen Dwight Reid Educational Foundation. Published by Heldref Publications, 4000 Albemarle Street, N.W., Washington, D.C. 20016. Copyright © 1970.

"Smokers' Rights Campaign Suffers from Lack of Dedicated Recruits." Reprinted by permission of *The Wall Street Journal.* Copyright © 1988 by Dow Jones & Company, Inc. All rights reserved worldwide.

"Taking on the Tobacco Institute; 'Other People's Smoke': Round Two." March 15, 1987. Copyright © 1987 by The New York Times Company. Reprinted by permission.

Turcol, Thomas. "Fairfax Restaurants Warm to Smoking Rules." April 20, 1986. Copyright © 1986 by *The Washington Post.* Reprinted by permission.

Excerpted with permission from "Nonsmokers: Time to Clear the Air" by C. Everett Koop, *Readers Digest,* April, 1987. Copyright © 1987 by The Readers Digest Association, Inc.

Library of Congress Cataloging-in-Publication Data

Allen, Steve, 1921–
  The passionate nonsmoker's bill of rights: the first guide to enacting nonsmoking legislation/Steve Allen and Bill Adler, Jr.
    p.   cm.
  Includes bibliographies and index.
  ISBN 0-688-06295-4
  1. Antismoking movement—United States. 2. Cigarette habit—United States. 3. Smoking—United States—Prevention. I. Adler, Bill, 1956–   . II. Title.
HV5763.A44   1989
362.2'967'0973—dc20   89-33857
                                                                             CIP

Printed in the United States of America

1 2 3 4 5 6 7 8 9 10

BOOK DESIGN BY MANUELA PAUL

From Steve Allen:

To Jayne, who never smoked again after she learned
that it displeased me

From Bill Adler, Jr.:

To Peggy, who is my fresh air

Foreword
by Steve Allen

Breathing is a very popular thing to do.

Anne Morrow Donley,
executive director,
Virginia GASP

Because I am a readily recognized public figure, it's hard to say whether it is easier, or more difficult, for me to assert myself in a situation where, in a public place, someone else's smoking louses up the air I'm breathing. Some years ago it occurred to me that to avoid awkward face-to-face confrontations it might be reasonable to have some business-card-size notes printed up, carrying the following message:

Dear Smoker:
    Perhaps it hasn't occurred to you that the smoke from your cigarette or cigar is at this moment offending a number of people around you. In any event, I'm sure I'm not alone in wishing that you would control your urge to smoke until you're once again out on the street.
    Thank you for your consideration of this request.

Sincerely,
A Nonsmoker

I had a hundred of the cards printed and carried a dozen or so of them in my wallet, ready to ask a maître d', waiter, or other employee to hand-deliver them to whatever thoughtless smokers I might encounter. For several months I found no occasion to distribute the cards, or at least no situation in which there was another person I could ask to make the delivery for me. But while at a good restaurant in Tokyo one evening, with my family, I was suddenly disturbed, in mid-meal, by the bitter, hideously unpalatable aroma of a really rotten cigar. "Aha," I said to myself, actually aloud. "I've got to send one of those cards over to that table."

I summoned a waiter, who fortunately spoke English, and said, "Do you see that gentleman at that table creating the clouds of cigar smoke?"

"Yes, sir," the waiter said.

"Good," I said. "Would you please hand him this card?"

Jayne, our sons, and I temporarily forgot about the matter since we were engrossed in conversation on another subject. Suddenly the relative quiet of the room was shattered by a roar of laughter. When I turned I saw that the semi-hysterical one was the man with the cigar who, it developed, had recognized me when he came into the restaurant. "Steve Allen, you crazy bastard," he said, good-naturedly enough. "You *would* do a nutty thing like this."

Since he was obviously prepared to be affable, I took the occasion to say, "Thanks for laughing it up but I really wasn't kidding. The smoke from your cigar is making it unpleasant for us here because we're still eating."

At that point a bit of the friendliness disappeared but I'm pleased to report that the stranger said, "Well, okay, if you insist."

The point of the story is that nonsmokers who care passionately about their freedom to breathe relatively unpolluted air will have to be either creative, socially aggressive, or both since many smokers are totally thoughtless.

Another method I employ is based on the premise that some smokers, who may be concentrating on other matters, literally are not aware that they are offending those around them and that, if they are somehow made aware of the trouble they are causing, they will be decent enough to snuff out their cigarettes, pipes, or cigars. One effective way of communicating a negative reaction to them is simply to be very obvious in waving a napkin, menu, or newspaper in front of one's face. The vigorous movement itself will generally attract the smoker's attention, or if his back is to you, the attention of others in his party. This method doesn't always work, I'm sorry to report, but in about 30 percent of the cases it does the trick.

Even hopelessly addicted smokers are willing to cooperate with airlines' rules and regulations if they are seated in a no-smoking section of the plane. Unfortunately, there are always a few exceptions. Some of them may just be seized by momentary absentmindedness. Others, I'm sure, know perfectly well that they're not supposed to smoke but perhaps figure that if no one complains they will be permitted to get away with it. Accordingly, whenever I detect clouds of smoke in a no-smoking section of the plane, I immediately call a flight attendant and say, "I may be mistaken, but it seems to me that there's an awful lot of smoke in the air, considering that this is a no-smoking section. Are you quite sure that no one in this area is smoking?"

The flight attendants are invariably helpful at such moments. They conduct a brief walking-and-looking tour and on rare occasions come back and say, "Thank you, Mr. Allen, for bringing that to our attention. We did discover one passenger smoking. The cigarette has now been put out."

While airlines, restaurants, and other corporate entities have all too begrudgingly and belatedly given consideration to the rights of nonsmokers, nothing short of the outright elimination of the practice can really balance the scales of justice between the two contending parties. The reason is that nothing I breathe in or out on an airplane can offend any other passenger, whereas the smoke exhaled or left to arise from cigarettes does ruin the air in every part of the plane, even that laughingly called the "no-smoking" section.

While it is true that the physical act of smoking is not permitted in these designated spaces, they could not possibly be truly smokefree areas for the simple reason that smoke drifts freely into them. The same thing is true, of course, of restaurants and other enclosed spaces.

The massive amount of utterly convincing medical evidence has, quite properly, moved the long-standing debate about the issue away from the area of assumption and speculation and into the realm of statistics and facts. But oddly enough, now that it is possible to speak authoritatively about emphysema, asthma, pneumonia, and allergic reactions, not to mention lung cancer, one rarely any longer hears much about the reason that occasioned the debate in the first place. And that is, quite simply, that millions of nonsmokers find the smell of tobacco unpleasant and, in extreme cases, nauseating. Those of us who consider such odors unpleasant, therefore, would still be protesting our treatment at the hands of smokers, even if the most outrageous claims of the tobacco companies were absolutely valid and no great physical harm resulted from the inhalation of smoke.

I have been biased against cigarettes, and their smoke, since infancy. Fortunately for me, but most unfortunately for my mother, she was a heavy smoker throughout most of her adult life. Since children often find the smell of cigarettes offensive, some of my earliest recollections involve waving my hands in front of my face to try to dissipate the foul-smelling fumes of my mother's cigarettes. When I was a few years older, and aware of the social factor of shame, I was often humiliated by the fact that not only did my mother smoke, something relatively rare among women during the 1920s and 1930s, but she compounded the crime by smoking on the street, or, indeed, anywhere it suited her pleasure to smoke. My mother naturally had her share of virtues but her inability to free herself of the compulsive addiction to smoking was a barrier between us throughout life. In her later years, when I would go to her apartment for a visit, the premises invariably smelled like one enormous ashtray and, as I arrived, she would dutifully empty such trays as were filled, in the vain hope that that would purify the atmosphere. Needless to say, the last dozen or so years of her life were spent in endless bouts of spitting, hacking, and coughing. A heart attack carried my mother away.

Among men and women who find the smell of cigarettes offensive, there is no way of knowing how many budding romances were early discouraged by the fact that an otherwise attractive member of the opposite sex was discovered to be a heavy smoker. I shall never forget the occasion, one New Year's Eve in Chicago long ago, when, at the stroke of midnight, all the other young couples observed the long-standing custom of sharing a kiss. I was willing to do the same; unfortunately the young lady in question had spent the previous few minutes smoking. Being involved in an animated conversation I had not paid particular attention to the fact of her smoking, but when she put her arms around my neck and gave me a warm kiss I was not stimulated, as I might otherwise have been, but was repulsed by the strong odor of burned tobacco on her breath.

*   *   *

While I did not become an antismoker because of personal family tragedy, smoking nevertheless has caused suffering to those close to me. My mother, as I said earlier, was hopelessly addicted to nicotine and the ritual of its daily use. It was therefore no surprise that she spent the last few years of her life with a constant, tremendously loud hacking cough, which not only caused her great discomfort but did not set too well with the many strangers around her in restaurants, theaters, and other public places. My half-brother, Young Smith, an attorney who lived in the south, also suffered years of impaired breathing because of his heavy smoking. Indeed on a couple of occasions when I visited him and his family, who had been alerted by my secretary to my own allergic reaction to cigarette and cigar smoke, poor Young, even though he wished to accommodate me, simply lacked the willpower to do so, so that the few days I shared his living quarters were decidedly uncomfortable, and partly sleepless, so heavily did the odor of his smoke permeate the premises. My wife Jayne's brother Frank, in his late years a judge of the Superior Court in Los Angeles, was most of his life a two-packs-a-day man and hence contracted lung cancer, to the surprise of no one in his family, and spent the last years of his life in dreadful suffering.

Steve Allen
Van Nuys, California

"CARELESS SMOKER"
Anti-Smoking Country and Western Song

Careless smoker, we've lost another motel.
Careless smoker, we've lost a million trees.
Careless smoker, we've lost another hotel.
Careless smoker, won't you stop it, please?

Because of you too many children will die,
From just one cigarette you left to burn.
Because of you a thousand mothers will cry.
Careless smoker, won't you ever learn?

You like to think that you're as tough as they come,
But most folks think you're really kinda dumb.

Careless smoker, see the people jump to their death.
See the flames climbing to the mountain-top.
Careless smoker, we can hardly catch our breath.
Careless smoker, when are you gonna stop?

Mister Smoker, there are widows lonely tonight,
'Cause you left a cigarette on some old shelf.
Careless smoker, don't you know that ain't right?
But you won't think of anybody but yourself.

Air pollution, it comes wherever you go,
And you make people lose their appetite.
Thoughtless smoker, there's so much you ought to know
about those lonesome sirens in the night.

Now you know that arson is a terrible crime.
Because of all the lives that it will take.
But careless smoker, without reason or rhyme
You leave death and destruction in your wake.

Meadowlane Music, ASCAP. Words and music by Steve Allen

Acknowledgments

Many people and organizations contributed their time, research and support for the three years that went into writing *The Passionate Nonsmoker's Bill of Rights*. We are grateful to them, for this book would have been impossible without their support. In return, we only hope that what we have written will help our friends, families, and colleagues get smokefree air wherever they are.

We thank Anne Morrow Donley, Tony Schwartz, Ahron Leichtman, Michele Kling, John Banzhaf, Ron Davis, Athena Mueller, Julia Carol, Noel McAfee, Ilene Freed, Patrick Reynolds, Dr. John H. O'Hara, Dr. Alan Blum, Carol Dana, and Marta Vogel.

The organizations that helped us immeasurably are the Surgeon General's Office on Smoking and Health, the American Lung Association, the American Cancer Society, the American Heart Association, Action on Smoking and Health (ASH), Americans for Nonsmokers' Rights, Citizens Against Tobacco Smoke, Doctors Ought to Care, the Tobacco Product Liabilities Project, Washingtonians for Nonsmokers' Rights, Virginia GASP, Bowie GASP, New Jersey GASP, GASP of Massachusetts, New York GASP, American Society of Internal Medicine, American Medical Association, American Academy of Pediatrics, and Group Health Cooperative of Puget Sound.

Many other people played a vital role in the creation of this book. *The Passionate Nonsmoker's Bill of Rights* was Bill Adler, Sr.,'s idea. Doug Stumpf, Senior Editor, and Jared Stamm, Assistant Editor, two of William Morrow's finest, guided this book along during its many phases. The unsung heroes of many books are the copy editors; in our case we are indebted to Robbie Capp for her incredible and painstaking attention to detail.

Contents

CONTENTS

Introduction

There is growing evidence that smoking has pharmacological . . . effects that are of real value to smokers.

Joseph F. Cullman III,
former president of Philip Morris,
Annual Report to Stockholders, 1962

Few social causes have grown as swiftly as the nonsmokers' rights
movement.

Nonsmokers' rights in the 1980s are gaining the same kind of
prominence, and having the same effects, as the antismog efforts had
in the early 1970s. Thanks to nonsmokers' rights legislation, people
are breathing cleaner, safer air.

Nonsmokers' rights laws—also called nonsmokers' health laws, and
clean air laws—are spreading across the country. Currently forty-one
states have some kind of restriction on smoking in public places.
Thirty-three states bar smoking on trains, buses, and subways;
seventeen states prohibit smoking in the workplace. Eight hundred
cities and towns ranging in size, geography, and culture from New
York City to Aspen, Colorado, to Somerville, Massachusetts, have
passed nonsmokers' rights laws. Some of these, like New York
State's, are very strong, others like the District of Columbia's, limit
smoking only in a few areas. Only eight states don't have any kind of
nonsmokers' rights laws: Alabama, Illinois, Louisiana, Missouri,
North Carolina, Tennessee, Virginia, and Wyoming.

In 1973 Arizona became the first state to pass nonsmokers' rights
legislation. Tobacco smoke was declared a public nuisance and

dangerous to health in elevators, indoor theaters, art museums, lecture and concert halls, public buses, school buildings, rest rooms, and public waiting areas of medical facilities.

But many places aren't waiting for a law to implement nonsmokers' rights: 54 percent of U.S. employers have some kind of no-smoking policy, including the Boeing Company, IBM, Connecticut Mutual Life Insurance, General Motors, L.L. Bean, and Campbell Soup. No smoking is reasonable, responsible, and the American way.

There are now over one hundred nonsmokers' rights groups across the country. It is a powerful movement.

Why has this movement come about? Perhaps the rapid growth of the nonsmokers' rights effort is a result of an increasing interest in health and fitness; perhaps it is an extension of antagonism toward the tobacco industry, which advertises a deadly product with the slogan "Alive with pleasure." Perhaps it's an evolutionary step: After outdoor air pollution was attacked, alleviated, and thousands of lives spared each year as a result, the next frontier could only be indoor air pollution. Or perhaps the nonsmokers' rights movement is a consequence of well-written, well-researched scientific studies that can't be ignored and that say, "Passive smoking causes disease." Whatever the mix of causes, there's no denying that the nonsmokers' rights movement has affected the lives of millions of Americans—for the better. But nonsmokers' rights still have a long way to go.

Why is this movement so large and so powerful? Two hundred million nonsmokers in the United States have grown tired of inhaling others' cigarette smoke. We've listened to the Surgeon General, the National Academy of Sciences, and other scientific and medical groups and we're concerned about the dangers of passive smoke. We don't want to be involuntary smokers because we don't want to become unwitting victims of lung cancer or emphysema. We choose not to smoke cigarettes and that means not breathing others' smoke.

Passive smoking is very dangerous. It can be deadly. One study by James Replace of the Environmental Protection Agency and A.H. Lowrey of the Naval Research Laboratory estimates that between five hundred and five thousand nonsmokers die each year *of lung cancer alone* from exposure to cigarette smoke. Emphysema, eye irritation, allergic reactions—and in children, reduced lung function, bronchitis, and increased incidence of pneumonia—these are some of the known perils of involuntary smoking. Substances such as carbon monoxide, polonium-210, hydrogen cyanide, nicotine, and dimethylnitrosamine permeate sidestream smoke.

What is passive smoking? Passive smoking is breathing in smoke against one's will. It is involuntarily smoking a cigarette. It is wrong.

Simply segregating smokers and nonsmokers does not eliminate the danger. Hundreds of sidestream smoke's microscopic particles and gasses freely drift through airliner cabins, office buildings, restaurants, and other enclosed spaces. Ventilation and air conditioning systems aren't designed to restrain the movement of these toxic chemicals. Secondhand smoke creates a cloud of indoor air pollution that grows larger as the day grows longer.

Freedom from tobacco smoke is a reasonable request, a necessary request. After all, 77 percent of all adults, including 64 percent of smokers, support no smoking around nonsmokers according to a 1987 Gallup Survey. There's hardly an issue on which so many Americans agree. And yet, there is tremendous opposition against the goal of protecting nonsmokers' health, almost all of it instigated by the cigarette companies and the Tobacco Institute.

Wherever there's a campaign to enact nonsmokers' rights, you'll find tobacco's representatives. They will be there with smooth tongues, fat wallets, and a menagerie of falsehoods to dispense about nonsmokers' rights. They will call the Surgeon General's report on passive smoking and health "a political document," insist that neither mainstream smoking nor involuntary smoking has been proven harmful, and proclaim that nonsmokers are really just "a few thousand fanatics."

Fighting for nonsmokers' rights isn't easy, but the victories are growing. Almost every week a town or county enacts some kind of nonsmokers' rights law because people's hearts—and lungs—say it's the right thing to do.

The nonsmokers' rights movement has many leaders. In the forefront of this battle are the American Cancer Society, American Lung Association, and American Heart Association, along with other powerful organizations such as Action on Smoking and Health (ASH), which fought for and won no-smoking sections on airplanes, Americans for Nonsmokers' Rights, and Citizens Against Tobacco Smoke. Prominent individuals including Larry Hagman, media expert Tony Schwartz, Yul Brynner (through a videotape being shown after his death), Sam Donaldson, Patrick Reynolds (grandson of R.J. Reynolds's founder), and Bob Keeshan (Captain Kangaroo) are also spearheading the nonsmokers' rights movement. Dozens of other medical groups, civic organizations, politicians, and businesses are fighting for nonsmokers' health legislation.

Ten years ago, few workplaces and few restaurants had no-smoking areas. Airplanes and buses offered no-smoking sections in the front, but by the end of a trip, every seat felt like it was in a smoking section. But a lot has happened over the past decade.

In 1987 the General Services Administration, the custodian of 6,900 federal buildings, barred smoking in all of the facilities it oversees. This affected about a million federal workers.

The United States Armed Forces prohibited smoking at most of its facilities in 1986. The order is part of a "health promotion" program instituted by then Secretary of Defense Caspar Weinberger.

Smoking is now prohibited on all domestic flights of less than two hours. (Northwest Airlines decided that *all* its domestic flights would be no-smoking.)

New York State's nonsmokers' rights law, which went into effect May 7, 1986, is among the most comprehensive in the nation. The law bans smoking in most indoor public places such as enclosed bus and train stations, shopping malls, theaters, arenas, hotel lobbies, taxicabs, schools, banks, hospitals, museums, and retail stores. (But not in tobacco stores, or at social functions such as weddings, parties, or public conventions.) Employers must provide smokefree working spaces for employees who want them. Restaurants with fifty or more seats must have a separate dining area that is large enough to satisfy the wants of nonsmokers. New York State Health Commissioner David Axelrod said the regulations "will save tens of thousands of lives."

Beverly Hills, California, requires separate smoking and no-smoking sections in restaurants, as well as air filtration systems. Palo Alto, California, and Aspen, Colorado, along with other cities prohibit smoking where food is served.

Cambridge, Massachusetts, banned smoking in most public places March 9, 1986. And the law is working superbly.

In the face of a multimillion-dollar tobacco industry lobbying campaign, it took San Francisco two tries to pass its comprehensive nonsmokers' rights legislation. But now workers in offices, patrons at restaurants, visitors in hospitals, and riders of public transportation are no longer involuntary smokers.

Nassau County, New York, and Fairfax, Virginia, both have regulations requiring restaurants to set aside at least 50 percent of their seats for nonsmokers. Many restaurants report that the no-smoking sections are continually filled.

The nonsmokers' rights movement is not an attempt to reform smokers. It doesn't seek to ban cigarettes or revive prohibition. Nonsmokers don't see smokers as a problem or even an issue; it's the sidestream smoke that's troublesome. Virtually all nonsmokers have friends and relatives who smoke, and would love for them to quit, but the nonsmokers' rights movement has nothing to do with that. While nonsmokers care about the health of their friends and relatives, the objective of the nonsmokers' rights campaign is to protect our own health. It is a personal health campaign.

Efforts to protect nonsmokers are moving forward on numerous fronts. Smoking may be banned in all federal buildings. It may be banned on all domestic airline flights. More states may propose separate smoking and no-smoking sections in restaurants, and require employers to take the rights of nonsmokers into consideration in the workplace. Smoking may be banned in hospitals and high schools. Taxicab passengers may be able to ask their drivers not to smoke, and drivers may be able to request that their passengers not smoke. Airport lounges and railroad waiting rooms could become off-limits to smokers. All of this may happen in the not-too-distant future. But not without more work.

On the legal front, there has already been one case where a tobacco company was found guilty of contributing to a smoker's death. This suit, *Cipollone* v. *Liggett & Myers, Philip Morris, and Lorillard,* was the first time a jury decided that tobacco smoking caused a smoker's death. There will be more legal verdicts against cigarette companies in the coming years; there may eventually be one in which cigarettes are found to be the cause of a nonsmoker's wrongful death.

While these bills and law suits don't directly address the concerns of the nonsmokers' rights movement, they are predicated on an intense desire to eliminate America's number-one health menace—cigarettes. Each year tobacco takes a terrible toll: Over 350,000 smokers and thousands of nonsmokers die needlessly.

The tobacco industry is a $40 billion-a-year business. It is tremendously profitable. Cigarette companies control not only the production of tobacco products, but own a broad range of subsidiaries including

Miller beer, My-T-Fine pudding, Napa Valley wineries, Vermont Maid syrups, General Foods, Swingline staples, and Saks Fifth Avenue. Each year cigarette companies spend $2 billion promoting their products. And they spend whatever it takes to thwart nonsmokers' health laws, despite the fact that the majority of smokers and nonsmokers want these laws. In researching and writing this book, we have become convinced that the major—and perhaps only—barrier to nonsmokers' rights laws is the tremendous power of the seven tobacco conglomerates. Smokers are usually willing to concede no-smoking sections and to accommodate nonsmokers in many ways. But the cigarette industry, usually through its Washington lobbying arm, the Tobacco Institute, doesn't believe that nonsmokers should be able to protect their health. The Tobacco Institute pretends to speak for smokers, claiming that nonsmokers' health laws would infringe on the "rights" of smokers. Only in the bizarre world of tobacco, could an organization claim to represent people and at the same time promote a product that kills them.

Is Smoking a Right?

Cigarette smoking is not a right. Not legally and certainly not ethically. The Constitution does not grant people the right to smoke. Just the opposite, the Constitution empowers the Congress and the states to act to protect the health of their citizens, and this includes protecting people from involuntary tobacco smoke. Most states and localities that have enacted laws to protect the rights of nonsmokers say that when there is a conflict between someone who wants to smoke and someone who wants clean air, the rights of the nonsmoker prevail. When there is a conflict between smokers and nonsmokers, especially in the workplace, courts have uniformly sided with nonsmokers. *There are no laws and no court decisions that proclaim the right to smoke.*

Smoking is a limited privilege, like spitting, throwing out garbage, listening to loud music, and drinking alcohol in public places. Citizens have the right to do these things so long as they do not bother or harm other people. The so-called right to smoke is a bogus notion, a fallacious fantasy created by the cigarette companies who want smokers to believe that others are out to take away their "rights."

Rights are indeed precious to Americans—and it's shameful when the tobacco companies twist the meaning of constitutional rights.

Cigarettes are a product, an element of the economy. They are a *thing*. There's no kinship between tobacco and freedom of assembly, freedom of speech, due process, or any constitutional guarantee. Tobacco is not like newspapers, protest demonstrations, a jury trial, civil rights, equal opportunity in work, or writing letters to members of Congress. The government has always had the authority to regulate or ban products. Cigarettes may be subject to taxation, licensing, health and safety standards, trade restrictions, recall for defectiveness, and fair advertising restrictions. Philosophically and legally there's no distinction between cigarettes or toaster ovens, automobile tires, candy, children's toys, and medicines.

The government has an important obligation to protect the life and health of Americans. Automobile speed limits, truck brakes, electrical wiring standards, prescription drug effectiveness, eyeglass lens strength, airplane inspections—these all fall under government regulations because of the government's duty to ensure the health and safety of its citizens. Sometimes it takes a long while before the government becomes active in an arena, as it did with certain food additives. And as with involuntary smoking. Government—that is, Congress and the states—is not perfect.

Cigarettes may be a legal consumer product, but they have a special attribute: They produce disease. If invented today, tobacco would never reach the market; it's simply too deadly. Cigarettes happen to be legal for a variety of reasons including that millions of Americans are addicted to them, the tobacco industry is rich and powerful, and cigarettes have been around for a long time. Perhaps they should be banned—or perhaps the officers of the cigarette companies ought to be imprisoned for producing and promoting a product that kills 350,000 users and at least 5,000 innocent bystanders a year. But banning cigarettes and convicting the people who make them is an issue for another book.

There's a related issue involved here: morality. Is it ethical to push a disease-producing, addictive product like cigarettes? Smoking cigarettes is one thing—nobody's arguing that individuals should not have the privilege of indulging in self-destructive activities. But enthusiastically encouraging people to engage in perilous behaviors is wrong. It's evil. Imagine for a moment that a parent or school teacher said to a fifteen-year-old, "Go ahead son, smoke cigarettes. Here's a couple of packs to start. I hope you like them and that you pick up the smoking habit." Outrage would be the response! Yet that's what the cigarette companies and the Tobacco Institute are doing. They are getting paid to bring smokers (and nonsmokers) closer to death. There's a tremendous difference between *choosing* to smoke (if in fact an informed choice can be made in the face of $2 billion a year in advertising) and someone *pushing* cigarettes. The tobacco industry and drug pushers share the same soul.

Also immoral is the Tobacco Institute's pretense of representing the interests of cigarette smokers. It does not. Sixty-two percent of smokers disagree with the Institute's position on not separating smokers from nonsmokers, and 87 percent of smokers want to quit. That image—being the spokesperson for America's smokers—is important for the Institute's credibility. But that image is a misrepresentation, mere smoke and mirrors. It's also perverse: Cigarettes kill and the Tobacco Institute is promoting cigarettes. How can the Institute represent people it's helping to kill? The Tobacco Institute is paid for by the cigarette manufacturers; that's whose interest the Institute represents.

Unfortunately, there is a conflict between smoking and people who want to breathe safe air. But as someone once remarked, your right to make a fist ends where my nose begins. Smokers' right to smoke stops where my lungs begin.

CHAPTER 1

The Power of Cigarette Companies and Cigarette Advertising

Exchange between Dr. Richard Manning, vice-president for Research and Development of U.S. Tobacco, and George Braly, attorney for the plaintiffs, during a trial in which U.S. Tobacco was accused of causing fatal mouth cancer in an eighteen-year-old boy:

Question (Braly): What is the range of nicotine found in tobacco?
Answer (Manning): I don't know.
Q: Did you tell the jury you are a tobacco chemist?
A: Yes, sir . . .
Q: No information on that subject?
A: No.

Later . . .
Q: What are carcinogens?
A: What do you mean by carcinogens?
Q: Doctor, my question is what are carcinogens?
A: I really don't know what you mean by carcinogens.
Q: I will tell you what I understand the word *carcinogen* to mean is something that causes cancer. Do you understand it any differently?
A: It causes cancer in what, sir?

Q: Animals.
A: What is cancer in animals? I am an organic chemist. I am not a pathologist. I am not an oncologist, I am not a medical doctor, and, no, I cannot answer that question because I don't know.

Still later . . .
Q: Is there anybody that works for the United States Tobacco Company that knows more about this particular subject of carcinogens than you do?
A: I didn't say I knew about this particular subject of carcinogens . . . Is your question, "Is there somebody that knows more than nothing?"
Q: About carcinogens.
A: I don't know.
Q: So if there is such a person that works for the U.S. Tobacco Company, you don't have any idea who it is?
A: Correct.
Q: And you admit to this jury that you know nothing about that subject?

Later, after Manning's attorney interjected . . .
Q: My question was didn't you just tell the jury that you didn't know of anybody in the company that knew more than nothing about carcinogens?
A: I think you are telling me I just said that.
Q: I am asking you, didn't you just say that a few minutes ago?
A: Right now I don't remember.

If you want to do battle in behalf of nonsmokers' rights, you have to know about the power of the tobacco companies. You have to know how they manipulate, cajole, and even coerce people and organizations. You have to know about the kind of money they willingly spend. Which means you have to know about cigarette advertising.

Advertising

Cigarette companies have two potent weapons on their side: The first is the addictive power of nicotine. The second is advertising. Advertising coaxes nonsmokers into the world of tobacco with sensual seductions and bold promises, and nicotine, along with more advertising, holds them in a psycho-physiological prison.

What the tobacco industry has had to say about advertising sheds much light on how they distort facts and lie to the public. It provides a quick lesson in how the cigarette companies practice the art of propaganda.

The Big Lie: Cigarette Advertising Doesn't Cause People to Smoke

The cigarette companies have had a century to perfect their advertising craft, and a century to perfect their denials about the effectiveness of advertising. The lie, one of tobacco's biggest, is that:

> The cigarette advertising of the Institute's member companies is brand advertising. It is designed to prompt smokers to switch brands or keep them loyal to the brands they already smoke. It does not *cause* smoking . . .
>
> *Horace R. Kornegay,*
> *chairman, the Tobacco Institute,*
> *testimony to the Subcommittee*
> *on Health and the Environment,*
> *U.S. House of Representatives,*
> *August 1, 1986*

Only a chowderhead would believe that cigarette advertising isn't designed to attract new smokers. Can anybody accept that the cigarette companies are not interested in encouraging people to smoke? It's a ludicrous notion. Cigarette companies are in the business of selling cigarettes—as many as they can. But the Tobacco Institute has to defend itself somehow, even if its only defense is made of paper-mâché lies.

The Tobacco Institute says that cigarette advertising is designed only to get smokers to switch brands. Really? Each year the cigarette companies spend over $2 billion in advertising,[1] some $8 for every American. Each year only 10 percent of smokers switch brands; this translates into a $2 billion shift in revenue.[2] Does anyone believe the industry's argument that cigarette companies spend $2 billion a year to earn $2 billion? Of course not.

Mr. Kornegay likes to make this analogy: "[Cigarette advertising] does not *cause* smoking any more than soap advertising causes people to bathe or detergent advertising causes people to wash their clothes." While it's impossible to quantify the effects of advertising, all consumer ads cause people to buy specific products that they've never owned before. Anybody in the advertising business will tell you that. But you don't even have to ask—just look at products like Pet Rocks, home computers, children's toys, sports cars, vacation spots, and compact disk players. Many, maybe most, people, are influenced to purchase these products because of advertising. Cigarettes are the most heavily advertised product in America, and the message that you should buy them sinks in, sinks in, sinks in, sinks in.

George Washington Hill, president of American Tobacco from 1925 to 1946 and one of the giants of the tobacco industry, said of cigarette advertising, "The impetus of those great advertising campaigns . . . built the cigarette industry."[3]

Spending on tobacco advertising increased four times in real dollars between 1971 and 1986, up from $200 million.

Philip Morris is the second-largest advertiser in the United States. RJR Nabisco is the fourth.[4]

The tobacco companies take their advertising very, very seriously. In 1988 Northwest Airlines banned smoking on all domestic flights. The advertising agency Northwest used to develop their smokefree flights advertisements was Saatchi & Saatchi, the agency that handles ads for some of RJR Nabisco's *noncigarette* products. After an eighteen-year relationship, RJR promptly fired Saatchi & Saatchi, which lost a $70 million account.

Newspapers and magazines believe that smoking can be caused by advertising—at least that's what they tell the cigarette companies. An advertisement by *The New York Times* in the *United States Tobacco and Candy Journal,* a trade publication of the tobacco industry, reminds cigarette companies, "Lifestyles are made, not born." *Newsweek*'s ad told cigarette companies they could "Light up your sales" with advertising in *Newsweek. Time* is another believer that cigarette advertising breeds smokers: "Where there's smoke . . . there's a hot market for cigarette advertisers in *Time.* The good news is certain demographic groups are hotter than ever; women, singles, 25–49-year-olds, and high school grads . . .''

Cigarette companies have to continue to attract new smokers because too many die too soon. The tobacco industry says there's no proof that smoking or involuntary smoking causes disease. Well, that's what they say. Here are the facts: Each year over 350,000 smokers die prematurely because of their cigarette addiction, and approximately another million quit (out of fifty million Americans who smoke). So just to keep even, the industry has to attract 1,350,000 new smokers every year! Notice that this is not optional: Merely to maintain their current level of sales, tobacco companies have to attract nearly one and a half million new smokers a year. And they succeed. Many smokers who quit, start again. And many people—mostly teenagers—who have never smoked, start each year. The tobacco companies are doing everything in their power to attract smokers. Nothing sneaky about that thought: Cigarette companies are in the business of doing more business.

We all know that cigarette advertising is banned from television. Right? Not exactly. Ever watch the Virginia Slims Tennis Tournament, or a soccer or football game? You'll see plenty of billboards for cigarettes posted around the stadium. Cigarette advertising is alive and well on television. According to *Business Week,* the purpose of sponsoring events ''is to get brands mentioned in news columns and on television, which bans cigarette advertising.''[5]

Cigarette Advertising Is Aimed at Specific Groups

Despite their denials that cigarette advertising is aimed at children and adolescents, cigarette companies do aim their advertising at specific markets—at women, blacks, blue-collar workers, upscale professionals (Yuppies and Preppies), Hispanics, *and especially children and adolescents.* An article in a 1986 issue of the industry's publication, the *United States Tobacco and Candy Journal,* reported that tobacco companies are coordinating advertising of specific brands with magazine readership.

But it's children that the tobacco companies' advertising affects most of all. Of course, the cigarette producers steadfastly deny that there is any attempt to enlist young smokers. Here's the most famous tobacco falsehood:

The cigarette industry long has taken the position that cigarette smoking is for adults only—adults who choose to smoke . . . In addition, the Institute and its member companies have sponsored a variety of advertisements encouraging the parents of young people to intercede with their children to prevent smoking. . . . The message of these advertisements perhaps is captured best by the headline of the center advertisement, which reads: "Do cigarette companies want kids to smoke? No. As a matter of policy. No. As a matter of practice. No. As a matter of fact. No!"

Tobacco company advertisement

How exactly do cigarette companies encourage teenagers not to smoke? They suggest that parents tell their children not to smoke (because we all know how effective parents are at controlling the behavior of adolescents). Then they print occasional notices in magazines and newspapers suggesting that kids not smoke. Hurrah for the cigarette companies!

Then what do the cigarette companies do for added measure? They put unchaperoned cigarette vending machines in restaurants, hotels, bus terminals, supermarkets—virtually everywhere. And they create advertisements which show smokers who are sexy, athletic, sophisticated—traits teenagers emulate.

And how effective are the tobacco companies at not getting teenagers to smoke? Of *all* smokers, 85 to 90 percent start smoking before they are nineteen years old! And 60 percent of all smokers start puffing away before they reach their fifteenth year! The average age at which someone is initiated into smoking is fourteen. Approximately 20 percent of all female and 16 percent of all male high school students are regular smokers.[6] And, most sadly, 22 percent of smokers start before they are nine.[7]

William Meyers wrote in his book about advertising, *The Image Makers,* "With most adult smokers already hooked on their favorite brands, the growth of individual tobacco companies depends on the uninitiated."

Said one fifteen-year-old girl, "It's easy for kids to get cigarettes. You just walk into any store and say, 'I'd like a pack of Marlboros.' You'll get them."[8] There's no disputing the fact that adolescents can buy cigarettes whenever they want.

But that's not all. If someone doesn't become a smoker by the time he is nineteen or twenty, chances are he will never smoke cigarettes. Only 10 percent of all smokers pick up the habit after they're nineteen. What this means is that *the cigarette companies must turn teenagers into smokers if they are to make money.* Cigarette companies have no choice: Unless they hook teenagers, they'll go out of business. Tobacco's future, to praraphrase an aphorism, is in our children. Tobacco companies *need* adolescents to maintain and expand their market.

The conservative magazine *The Economist* concluded: ''The main new market (for cigarettes) must be teenagers.''[9]

Cigarette advertisements appeal to adolescents—and that allure isn't accidental. A two-frame Benson & Hedges ad shows a woman smoking a cigarette sitting at a table in a restaurant with another woman who's not smoking. There's a man smoking at the table next to them. In the next picture the man and woman who are smoking are smiling seductively at each other. Or how about the Lucky Strike advertisement in which the attractive woman in dark sunglasses is saying ''Light my Lucky?'' The only adolescent boys that ad doesn't appeal to are the ones who don't see it. The Kool Milds advertisement with the cool-looking man and woman—he with a muscle shirt and leaning against a wall and she wearing a jean jacket with her foot on the front fender of a motor cycle—also enthralls the rebellious, adventurous, adolescent spirit and mind.

Suggest that advertising causes people to smoke and the cigarette companies jump up and down shouting ''Noooo, tobacco advertising only induces people to switch brands.'' Well, look at the brands of cigarettes most popular with children—Marlboro for instance, and then examine Marlboro ads. Then scan the advertisements for cigarettes that are not popular with children, such as Merit. You'll notice a major difference between the two and the difference is this: Cigarettes that children smoke are advertised in ways that appeal to adolescents. Different advertisements appeal to different sexes and age groups. One psychologist reported, ''Sixth-grade females identified more closely with the self-reliant Marlboro cowboy and the self-confident Salem man than with the fun-loving actress in the More ad or the nonconformist woman in the Golden Lights ad. This helps explain why nearly 60 percent of the thirteen- and fourteen-year-old girl smokers in Los Angeles and over 80 percent of the thirteen- and fourteen-year-old girl smokers in Minneapolis report smoking

Marlboro cigarettes.''[10] Over 50 percent of all teenage smokers smoke Marlboro.

And so on. Regardless of what the tobacco companies say their advertisements are supposed to do, these ads do influence children to buy cigarettes.

R.J. Reynolds sponsors fashion shows, rock concerts, country-music festivals, sports events including skiing and race car driving, and sports clothing with the cigarette-brand logos. All of these activities pique the interest of teenagers. So does *Moviegoer* magazine, which is chock full of cigarette ads and is aimed at the thirteen- to thirty-year-old audience, and which is distributed free at movie theaters in hundreds of cities.[11]

An advertising executive told Dr. Alan Blum, chairman of Doctors Ought to Care (DOC) and former editor of the *New York State Journal of Medicine*:

> When I worked for [a major New York advertising agency] we were trying very hard to influence kids who were fourteen years old to smoke. The entry age is fourteen. I was laughing on the outside and crying on the inside. My experience tells me never to believe any noble notions about advertising men— that they won't aim at kids. They will aim at whoever the client is and they have determined will sell the product. They do not care what the product is.[12]

Marketing & Research Counselors, Inc., was hired in 1975 to examine potential new buyers for Brown & Williamson's Viceroy and to create the best image for that cigarette. The report, sent to Ted Bates, Brown & Williamson's advertising agency, revealed how young smokers *and nonsmokers* could be wooed into smoking:

> For the young smoker, the cigarette is not yet an integral part of life, of day-to-day life, in spite of the fact that they try to project the image of a regular run-of-the-mill smoker. For them, a cigarette, and the whole smoking process, is part of the illicit pleasure category. . . . In the young smoker's mind a cigarette falls into the same category with wine, beer, shaving, wearing a bra (or *purposefully* not wearing one), declaration of independence, and striving for self-identity. For

the young starter, a cigarette is associated with introduction to sex life, with courtship, with smoking "pot," and keeping late studying hours . . .

Thus, an attempt to reach young smokers, starters, should be based, among others, on the following major parameters:

- Present the cigarette as one of the few initiations into the adult world.
- Present the cigarette as part of the illicit pleasure category of products and activities.
- In your ads create a situation taken from the day-to-day life of the young smoker but in an elegant manner have this situation touch on the basic symbols of the growing-up, maturity process.
- To the best of your ability (considering some legal con-straints) relate the cigarette to "pot," wine, beer, sex, etc.
- Don't communicate health or health-related points.[13]

Bob Keeshan, better known as Captain Kangaroo, summed up the cigarette companies' strategies well:

The tobacco industry's marketing strategies are textbook examples of how to sell. Young people are targeted, despite industry denials, and are told, over and over again, that smoking is healthy, sexy, and the fast road to growing up. The message for the "hurried generation" is in magazines, news-papers, on the public bus kids take to school. The message is transmitted through industry sponsorship of sporting events, rock concerts, and even cultural events. A young person must question, "How can the product be bad if it is associated with such good activities?" The industry attempts to make its product "healthy by association."[14]

Children simply do not have sufficient information about the health effects of cigarettes to make a "cost versus benefit" decision about smoking. They don't understand about emphysema, heart attacks, and lung cancer—diseases that are decades into their future. They are not informed about tobacco's addictiveness.

Once children start using cigarettes, the addictive power of nicotine takes over. In his 1988 report, the Surgeon General concluded that nicotine is a powerfully addictive substance: "Cigarettes and other forms of tobacco are addicting; Nicotine is the drug in tobacco that causes addiction."[15] Tobacco advertising combined with nicotine are a potent combination—a combination that children can't beat.

A producer at a New York radio station once explained to Tony Schwartz why the station did not run antismoking spots. It wasn't because of the income the station received from tobacco advertising, because advertising cigarettes on radio is banned. The reason was far more subtle:

> My concern in carrying any of these spots is that we do considerable business with Miller Beer [a Philip Morris subsidiary] and other companies with Philip Morris directly. Not with the cigarette side of it, but [with] companies that they're affiliated with. And I have some kind of a concern as to—would there be a backlash? No matter how covered it might be, we do a lot of business with 7-Up, Miller Beer, and General Foods . . . We probably do, for example, in excess of $300,000 a year on Miller Beer. That's a considerable amount of money which we wouldn't want to jeopardize . . . We may not get anything directly from Philip Morris, but, the [advertising] agencies that handle these accounts could certainly buy around a radio station.

That's the power of the tobacco companies.

NOTES

(1) According to the Federal Trade Commission, tobacco companies spent $2.5 billion on marketing in 1985.
(2) *The Economist,* July 26, 1986, p. 20.
(3) *Congressional Quarterly,* January 21, 1977.
(4) *Advertising Age.*

(5) *Business Week,* December 7, 1981, p. 65.

(6) Frank Palumbo, M.D., Director of the Child Ambulatory Services Department at Georgetown University Medical Department; Charles A. Lemaistre, M.D., president, American Cancer Society, testimonies before the U.S. House of Representatives, Committee on Energy and Commerce, Subcommittee on Health and the Environment, July 18, 1986.

(7) Tony Schwartz, testimony, U.S. House of Representatives, loc. cit.

(8) Keri Licht, *Tobacco and Youth Reporter,* Autumn 1988.

(9) *The Economist,* July 26, 1986, p. 20.

(10) William J. McCarthy, Ph.D., assistant research psychologist, University of California, testimony before the U.S. House of Representatives, loc. cit.

(11) Alan Blum, M.D., testimony before the U.S. House of Representatives, loc. cit.

(12) Ibid.

(13) Peter Taylor, *The Smoke Ring* (New York, New American Library, 1984), Citation from Document AO11345, Federal Trade Commission, pp. 200–201.

(14) Testimony before the U.S. House of Representatives, loc. cit.

(15) *The Health Consequences of Smoking: Nicotine Addiction,* a Report of the Surgeon General, May 1988, p. i.

CHAPTER 2

The Health Effects of Involuntary Smoking

"Nobody's banned chewing gum because twice last
year you got some stuck on your shoe."

The Tobacco Observer,
March 1987

One of the first warnings about the health effects of smoking was issued on October 22, 1954 by the American Cancer Society: "The . . . available evidence indicates an association between smoking, particularly cigarette smoking, and lung cancer." But another ten years were to pass until the dangers of mainstream smoking became widely known. In 1964 Surgeon General Luther Terry issued his now-historic report on smoking and health. Since then a gigantic number of studies—over fifty thousand—have defeated any doubt that smoking cigarettes can be deadly. Cigarettes are sleeping dragons that wait twenty or thirty years before revealing their awful and powerful teeth, ravishing and torturing the body with lung cancer, emphysema, heart disease, cancer of the mouth and tongue, and a host of other horrors. Death by smoking is painful and lingering.

Smoking cigarettes kills over 350,000 Americans each year. (Some studies say as many as 500,000 Americans die each year from smoking.)[1] That is more than the combined deaths from all of the following: alcohol, cocaine, AIDS, heroin, PCP, and automobile accidents. Tobacco-related illnesses result in 2.5 million deaths a year worldwide.[2] A typical smoker dies ten years earlier than her nonsmoking friends. A pack-and-a-half-a-day smoker is seventeen times more likely than a nonsmoker to die of bronchitis, emphysema, or lung cancer. More Americans die each year from holding cigarettes in their own hands than died at the hands of the Nazis in Word War II. If the angel of death has a physical form it is cigarettes.

As Surgeon General C. Everett Koop said, "If we woke up tomorrow morning knowing nothing about the health hazards of cigarettes, and suddenly *The New York Times, The Wall Street Journal,* and the *Los Angeles Times* said 350,000 people died last year from smoking, there would be rioting in the streets."[3]

Even the tobacco companies have long known that smoking cigarettes is dangerous, although they choose to keep this information from the public. These revelations came about during the *Cipollone* v. *Liggett, et al.* trial in 1988, when, for the first time, a cigarette company was held liable for the death of a smoker. One trial document showed that the Committee for Tobacco Research, formed in 1954 by the cigarette companies to combat rumors that smoking causes tumors, uncovered, and then suppressed, a study that linked smoking to cancer in hamsters.[4] Four years later the Tobacco Industry Research Committee, in an internal report, said, "Results . . . indicated that persons with severe or very severe emphysema would be better off to stop smoking."[5] The plaintiffs also disclosed a 1961 tobacco company memorandum that said, "There are biologically active materials present in cigarette tobacco. These are: a) cancer-causing [and] b) cancer promoting."[6] Another tobacco industry report in 1963 said, "Evidence is available which suggests that chronic smokers are more likely to develop disturbances of lipid metabolism, develop a greater incidence of coronary artery disease at a younger age, and manifest a higher incidence of coronary occlusion."[7]

Evidence that involuntary smoking is harmful is also medically clear and conclusive. According to the Surgeon General:

> 1. Involuntary smoking is a cause of disease, including lung cancer, in healthy nonsmokers.
> 2. The children of parents who smoke compared with the children of nonsmoking parents have an increased frequency of respiratory infections, increased respiratory symptoms, and slightly smaller rates of increase in lung function as the lung matures.
> 3. The simple separation of smokers and nonsmokers within

the same air space may reduce, but does not eliminate, the exposure of nonsmokers to environmental tobacco smoke.[8]

The National Academy of Sciences offers these statistics:

Among studies of various populations in Europe, Asia, and North America, the risk of lung cancer is roughly 30 percent higher for nonsmoking spouses of smokers than it is for nonsmoking spouses of nonsmokers. There is consistency among the studies in that all the studies individually include the 30 percent increased risk within the 95 percent confidence intervals.[9]

The Academy concludes that sidestream smoke causes approximately 2,400 lung cancer deaths a year.[10]

What We Know About Passive Smoking

It's worth probing a little deeper into the Surgeon General's and National Academy of Sciences' reports, for as revealing as their conclusions are, the details of these reports are even more disturbing. These reports, along with dozens of other studies, show that passive smoking is a clear and present danger, one that increases the more you are exposed to sidestream smoke.

Dr. Barbara S. Hulka, chairman of the University of North Carolina's Department of Epidemiology, and chair of the National Academy of Sciences' report on passive smoking, summarized the NAS and Surgeon General's reports:

Both reports concluded that nonsmokers who have been chronically exposed to passive smoke are at increased risk of cancer; that children of smoking parents have increased risk for lung cancer; that children of smoking parents have increased respiratory illnesses compared with children whose parents do not smoke; and that insufficient data exist for other diseases, such as cancer other than lung and cardiovascular diseases. The NAS report also found that passive smoking causes very real acute effects in many nonsmokers—largely through irritation of eyes, nose and throat. . . .We concluded that, taken as a whole, passive smoking does increase the risk of lung cancer in nonsmokers. Just because current studies are limited to spousal exposure in the home does not mean that other populations with similar exposures are not similarly affected.[11] *finish*

Medical research has established an important principle: *Once a substance is identified as a carcinogen or poison in a particular environment—such as asbestos or lead in buildings—it is understood to cause damage to human tissue in all environments.* In other words, there are no safe environments for tobacco smoke: It causes cancer in laboratory animals, in smokers, and in nonsmokers. Sidestream smoke in public places is a public health hazard.

It makes sense that involuntary smoking should be toxic: Sidestream smoke contains over four thousand chemicals, some of which are known carcinogens, others potent poisons. Sidestream smoke, in fact, contains more dangerous components than does mainstream tobacco smoke partly because mainstream smoke is filtered. The constituents of sidestream smoke fall into two categories: gases and particles. Both have their own insidious qualities: Gases, such as carbon monoxide, cannot be removed from the air with air-conditioning or other closed ventilation systems. Particles can be removed in part by sophisticated and vastly expensive ventilation systems, but they also lodge in the lungs of nonsmokers. Here's a short list of some of the nastier components of sidestream smoke:

GASES

CARBON MONOXIDE, a by-product of incomplete combustion, is a poison. It interferes with the ability of red blood cells to absorb oxygen; carbon monoxide's affinity for hemoglobin is three hundred times that of oxygen. CO forces oxygen to be expelled from the tissues, causing them to be asphyxiated. It deprives the brain and other vital organs of oxygen and can reduce alertness in concentrations as low as 0.01 percent. At levels of 0.4 percent carbon monoxide is fatal.

HYDROGEN CYANIDE is a poison most people have heard of in connection with execution of criminals. It interferes with cells' metabolism of oxygen, and in the doses found in cigarette smoke, hydrogen cyanide destroys cilia, the tiny hairs leading to the lungs that keep the lungs clean.

CARBON DIOXIDE acts like carbon monoxide in many ways, substituting itself for oxygen in the cells. It is dangerous, but not as toxic as carbon monoxide.

BENZOPYRENE 3.4 is a polycyclic hydrocarbon that causes cancer.

PARTICULATES

NICOTINE was discovered in 1828. It is a potent poison; forty to sixty milligrams will kill an adult. It is addictive, with properties similar to heroin and cocaine; children and teenagers may be particularly susceptible to nicotine addiction. Nicotine "and smoking exert effects on nearly all components of the endocrine and neuro-endocrine systems (including catecholamines, serotonin, cortico-steroids, pituitary hormones). Some of these endocrine effects are mediated by actions of nicotine on brain neurotransmitter systems (e.g. hypothalamic-pituitary axis). In addition, nicotine has direct peripherally mediated effects (e.g., on the adrenal medulla and the adrenal cortex)."[12]

DIMETHYLNITROSAMINE is one of the most potent carcinogens known. It produces cancer in all species tested and can cause cancer in as little as a single exposure.

POLONIUM-210 is a radioactive element found in mainstream and sidestream smoke. It causes cancer.

Sidestream smoke falls into a category of substances known as indoor air pollutants. Indoor air pollution can present a greater danger to health than outdoor air pollution, because indoor air contaminates are not diluted or expelled from interior environments. (Sometimes outdoor air pollution suffers a similar fate: Inversions, no wind, and surrounding mountains can prevent outdoor air pollution from being mixed with cleaner air and blown away.) In addition, people spend the majority of their time inside.

Passive Smoking and Children

The Surgeon General is especially concerned about the effects of involuntary smoking on children: Children, the youngest of whom don't even know what a cigarette is, are true involuntary smokers. They usually *can't* leave a room and aren't able to challenge a smoker. Although children are exposed to cigarette advertising, there's little chance that they've heard or read anything about the health dangers of passive smoking. The children who are at greatest risk are the ones who can't even read or talk: During the first two years of life, infants of parents who smoke are more likely than infants of nonsmoking parents to be hospitalized for bronchitis and pneumonia. Children whose parents smoke also develop respiratory symptoms more frequently, and they show small, but measurable differences on tests of lung function when compared with children of nonsmoking parents. Respiratory infections in young children of smokers may increase susceptibility to develop lung disease as an adult.[13]

The Surgeon General's 1986 report evaluated several studies on smoking and children. He found that children of smoking parents spend much more time in hospitals than children whose parents don't smoke. In one Israeli study that examined 10,672 children born between 1965 and 1968, researchers disovered that "infants, whose mothers, at a prenatal visit, reported that they smoked, had a 27.5 percent greater hospital admission rate for pneumonia and bronchitis than children of nonsmoking mothers." In another study (Rantakallio, 1978) 3,600 children were followed during their first five years. "The children of mothers who smoked had a 70 percent greater chance of hospitalization for a respiratory illness than the children of nonsmoking mothers."[14]

In addition to the deadly serious problems of pneumonia and bronchitis, children of smoking parents have many more incidences of coughs, phlegm, and wheezing. One retrospective study (McConnochie and Roghmann, 1984) found that "involuntary smoking was a significant predictor of current wheezing (odds ratio 1:9)."[15] Another study of 650 children aged five to ten years (Weiss et al. 1980), "significant trend in the reported prevalence of chronic wheezing with current parental smoking was found; the rates were 1.9 percent, 6.9 percent, and 11.8 percent for children with zero, one, and two parents who smoked, respectively."[16] The Surgeon General concludes:

> In summary, children whose parents smoke had a 30 to 80 percent excess prevalence of chronic cough or phlegm compared with children of nonsmoking parents. For wheezing the increase in risk varied from none to over sixfold among the studies reviewed. Many studies showed an exposure-related increase in the percentage of children with reported chronic symptoms as the number of parental smokers in the home increased.[17]

Children of smoking parents are damaged in other ways, too. Again the Surgeon General: "The available data demonstrate that maternal smoking reduces lung function in young children. However, the absolute magnitude of the difference in lung function is small on average. . . . However, some children may be affected to a greater extent, and even small differences might be important for children who become active cigarette smokers as adults."[18]

It also seems that infants whose mothers smoke while pregnant have a 50 percent higher risk of Sudden Infant Death Syndrome. A British study discovered that children born to women who smoked ten or more cigarettes a day were three to five months behind their peers in reading and math.[19] As the American Cancer Society put it, pregnant women who smoke are "smoking for two."

So seriously are children affected by tobacco, that if it weren't for bizarre legal and social consequences, smoking around children would be a form of child abuse.

Ear infections, including glue ear, otitis media, and middle ear problems are also more common among children of smoking parents.[20] These infections can be chronic and can lead to disease. Other problems, including nasal congestion, are also common among children exposed to sidestream smoke.

Passive Smoking and Adults

Well before there were any studies linking passive smoking and disease, people had a good idea that breathing cigarette smoke was not smart: A body reacting with burning eyes, coughing, headaches, nausea, is making a clear biological statement. No amount of tobacco flavoring and scents mollifies these reactions. Bodies put out these signs for good reasons: to warn their owners to avoid tobacco smoke.

These initial perceptions were eventually borne out by scientific studies. One of the first examinations of passive smoking and disease was written by James Replace of the Environmental Protection Agency and A.H. Lowrey of the Naval Research Laboratory. They estimated that passive smoking causes between five hundred and five thousand lung cancer deaths a year.[21] They found that deaths from involuntary smoking are two orders of magnitude higher than predicted for other cancer-causing agents which are regulated as hazardous air pollutants under the Clean Air Act.

Dr. Lawrence A. Meinert reported in *New Jersey Medicine* that nonsmokers exposed to cigarette smoke increase their risk of lung cancer by 25 percent over people who live and work in smokefree environments.[22] But even in the absence of lung cancer, nonsmokers exposed to tobacco smoke experience a decline in lung function.

In testimony before the U.S. Senate[23] Replace elaborated on his article, pointing out that passive smoking is an important issue because Americans spend an average of 90 percent of their time indoors. He emphasized that sidestream smoke is even more carcinogenic than mainstream smoke, and that his estimate of up to five thousand lung cancer deaths a year is a particularly disturbing figure because it represents "nearly one third of the annual lung cancer mortality in nonsmokers." In the typical U.S. office workplace, under average conditions of occupancy and ventilation, the tobacco-smoke-caused lung cancer risk to the nonsmoking office workers appears to be, depending on the ventilation, two hundred fifty to a thousand times the level of acceptable risk using standard federal guidelines for carcinogens in air or water or food.

A January 1986 editorial in the *American Review of Respiratory Disease* said of the Replace-Lowrey study, "Replace and Lowrey's figures remain the best current estimates of lung cancer deaths from passive smoking. Current epidemiologic data are sufficiently imprecise to be able to accurately distinguish between the estimate of five hundred or five thousand deaths per year. The higher figure seems a more plausible estimate from the current data. Future epidemiologic studies will allow revision of these estimates but are unlikely to dispute the basic nature of the association.''

More information about involuntary smoking becomes available all the time, and it's not good.

> Consider . . . the findings of one of the most extensive investigations to date on the effects of second-hand smoke on the health of women . . . conducted by Michael Martin, M.D., a clinical epidemiologist at the University of California at San Francisco. Dr. Martin and his associates looked into the medical histories of more than 7000 nonsmoking women between the ages of 30 and 59. His main finding: nonsmoking wives of current smokers were 3.4 times more likely to suffer heart attacks than wives of men who never smoked, and nearly twice as prone to heart attacks as wives of men who formerly smoked.[24]

One constituent of sidestream smoke that may have particularly damaging properties are radioactive particles, in particular polonium-210 and lead-210.[25] Dr. John H. O'Hara, Ph.D., points out:

> Recent studies suggest that tobacco smoke may be the major source of radioactive exposure to the majority of Americans. For example, Black, et al., have shown that approximately 7 percent of the radioactivity in tobacco is transferred to the mainstream smoke inhaled by the smoker, while 30 percent is transferred to sidestream smoke. Given that the radioactive exposure to large concentrations of secondhand smoke could result in nonsmokers' exposure exceeding the government-recommended maximum dosage . . . clinical and epidemiologic studies on animals and humans have shown strong positive correlations between the increased incidence of cancer and the increased dose exposure to radiation. In addition, these studies have shown a dramatic increase in cancer rates when the control groups were also exposed to tobacco smoke.[26]

More recent studies have found more relationships between sidestream smoke and lung cancer. A study released in 1985 that examined 134 nonsmoking women with lung cancer found that those who lived with a smoking husband had an increased lung cancer risk of between 13 and 31 percent. If the woman lived with a husband who smoked twenty or more cigarettes per day, her chances of contracting lung cancer were *twice as high as for the wife of a nonsmoker.*[27]

A Japanese study, called the Hirayama study after its author, examined 91,540 women between 1966 and 1979. The study found a 1.9 factor (nearly two times) increase in lung cancer rates for nonsmokers whose spouses smoked 20 or more cigarettes a day, and a 1.4 factor increase for incidence of lung cancer among spouses who smoked between 1 and 14 cigarettes a day. A Greek study conducted by Trichopoulos and colleagues looked at the effects of passive smoking on the lung cancer risk of 51 female lung cancer patients and 163 controls. Wives of husbands who smoked 21 or more cigarettes a day experienced a 2.5-fold lung cancer rate increase. Wives of men who consumed 1 to 20 cigarettes a day had a lung cancer incidence with a 1.9 factor increase above normal.

Cigarette smoke causes the death of nonsmokers in other, more direct ways. Each year over a thousand Americans are killed because of fires caused when cigarettes ignited bedding, upholstery, and furniture.[28] Approximately half that number—five hundred people—were not the smoker; they were killed because someone else caused the fire.

In too many ways, involuntary smoking is dangerous, and often deadly. The more studies that are conducted, the more we learn about the perils of passive smoke.

Constituents of Sidestream Smoke: Ratio of Mainstream Smoke (MS) to Sidestream Smoke (SS) in Nonfilter Cigarettes

Tobacco smoke contains four thousand known components, of which forty-eight are known carcinogens. Tar, one of these cancer-causing chemicals, is 70 percent higher in sidestream smoke than in mainstream smoke; benzopyrene is 3.4 times higher. There is no such thing as a "safe" level of exposure to tobacco smoke.[29]

The following is only a partial list of the dangerous materials found in sidestream smoke.

VAPOR PHASE CONSTITUENTS
SOURCE: SURGEON GENERAL'S REPORT, 1986

Substance	MS Range	SS–MS Range
Carbon monoxide	10–23 mg	2.5–4.7
Carbon dioxide	20–40 mg	8–11
Carbon sulfide	18–42 μg	0.03–0.13
Benzene	12–48 μg	10
Toluene	160 μg	6
Formaldehyde	70–100 μg	0.1–50
Acrolein	60–100 μg	8–15
Pyridine	16–40 μg	6.5–20
3-Methylpyridine	12–36 μg	3–13
3-Vinylpyridine	11–30 μg	20–40
Hydrogen cyanide	400–500 μg	0.1–0.25
Hydrazine	32 ng	3
Ammonia	50–130 μg	40–170
Methylamine	11.5–28.7 μg	4.2–6.4
Dimethylamine	7.8–10 μg	3.7–5.1
Nitrogen oxide	100–600 μg	4–10
N-Nitrosodimethylamine*	10–40 ng	20–100
N-Nitrosopyrrolidine*	6–30 ng	6–30
Formic acid	210–490 μg	1.4–1.6
Acetic acid	330–810 μg	1.9–3.6

PARTICULATE PHASE CONSTITUENTS
SOURCE: SURGEON GENERAL'S REPORT, 1986

Substance	MS Range	SS–MS Range
Particulate matter*	15–40 mg	1.3–1.9
Nicotine	1–2.5 mg	2.6–3.3
Anatabine	2–20 μg	0.1–0.5
Phenol	60–140 μg	1.6–3.0
Catechol	100–300 μg	0.6–0.9
Hydroquinone	110–300 μg	0.7–0.9
Aniline	360 ng	30
2-Toluidine	160 ng	19
2-Naphthylamine*	1.7 ng	30

* = Human or animal carcinogen

4-Aminobiphenyl*	4.6 ng	31
Benz(a)anthracene*	20–70 ng	2–4
Benzo(a)pyrene	20–40 ng	2.5–3.5
Cholesterol	22 μg	0.9
Y-Butyrolactone*	10–22 μg	3.6–5.0
Quinoline	0.5–2 μg	8–11
Harman	1.7–3.1 μg	0.7–1.7
N-Nitrosonornicotine*	200–3,000 ng	0.5–3
NNK*	100–1,000 ng	1–4
N-Nitrosodienthanolamine*	20–70 ng	1.2
Cadmium	100 ng	7.2
Nickel	20–80 ng	13–30
Zinc	60 ng	6.7
Polonium-210*	0.04–0.1 pCi	1.0–4.0
Benzoic acid	14–28 μg	0.67–0.95
Lactic acid	63–174 μg	0.5–0.7
Glycolic acid	37–126 μg	0.6–0.95
Succinic acid	110–140 μg	0.43–0.62

* = Human or animal carcinogen

NOTES

(1) *New Jersey Medicine,* February 1988, p. 102.
(2) "Health Experts Blast Promotion of U.S. Tobacco in Third World," *The Washington Post,* February 19, 1988, p. A6.
(3) Dr. C. Everett Koop, *This Week With David Brinkley,* March 27, 1988.
(4) "Opposing Health Claims Open N.J. Tobacco Trial," Morton Mintz, February 2, 1988, *The Washington Post,* p. E2.
(5) *Tobacco and Youth Reporter,* Autumn 1988, p. 10.
(6) "Expert: Tobacco Firms Knew Risk, Didn't Tell Public," Morton Mintz, February 5, 1988, *The Washington Post,* p. F1.
(7) S. Ballet, "Physiologic Basis for Prohibition Against Smoking," *Coronary Heart Disease,* quoted in the 1963 report of the Tobacco Industry Research Council.
(8) *The Health Consequences of Involuntary Smoking,* a report of the U.S. Department of Health and Human Services, 1986, p. 13.

(9) *Environmental Tobacco Smoke: Measuring Exposures and Assessing Health Effects,* National Academy Press (Washington, D.C., 1986), p. 7.

(10) Dr. C. Everett Koop, remarks at press conference releasing the 1986 Surgeon General's report on *The Health Consequences of Involuntary Smoking.*

(11) *The New York Times,* March 15, 1987, p. C12.

(12) *The Health Consequences of Smoking: Nicotine Addiction,* a Report of the Surgeon General, May 1988, p. 14.

(13) Surgeon General's 1986 report, p. 10.

(14) Ibid. pp. 42–43.

(15) Ibid. p. 47

(16) Ibid. p. 47.

(17) Ibid. p. 48.

(18) Ibid. p. 54.

(19) *Newsweek,* "Women Smokers: The Risk Factor," November 25, 1985, p. 76.

(20) NAS, op. cit., p. 274; The Surgeon General op. cit., p. 59.

(21) *Environment International,* Vol. 11, pp. 3–22.

(22) "Scientific Basis for Workplace Clean Air," *New Jersey Medicine,* p. 141.

(23) U.S. Senate Subcommittee on Civil Service, Post Office, and General Services, Committee on Governmental Affairs, September 30, 1985.

(24) Dr. C. Everett Koop, "Nonsmokers: Time to Clear the Air," *Reader's Digest,* April 1987, p. 112.

(25) Polonium-210 has a half-life of 138 days, and lead-210 has a half-life of 22 years.

(26) John H. O'Hara, Ph.D., "Radioactivity and cigarette smoke," Letter, *New York State Journal of Medicine,* December 1983.

(27) *The Washington Post,* February 5, 1986, health section, p. 7.

(28) *The Washington Post,* April 25, 1985, p. A21.

(29) *American Society of Internal Medicine,* "Facts on Passive Smoking," 1988.

CHAPTER 3

Starting a Nonsmokers' Rights Group

A Couple of Thoughts about Statistics from the Tobacco Institute:

You can prove anything with statistics.

> *Brennan Dawson,*
> *public relations officer,*
> *the Tobacco Institute,*
> *on* The Diane Rehm Show,
> *National Public Radio,*
> *December 18, 1986,*
> *commenting on the health*
> *effects of passive smoking*

If it is the intention of the antismoking advocates to stop people from smoking, then banning the ads won't do it . . . The smoking industry competes for brand switching. Statistics show that of the fifty-five million smokers, 90 percent of them usually stick to one brand. Another 10 percent will switch.

> *Brennan Dawson,*
> *public relations officer,*
> *the Tobacco Institute,*
> *the* Cincinnati Enquirer,
> *September 19, 1986*

If you want to enact nonsmokers' rights legislation in your state or municipality, a nonsmokers' rights group is the best way to begin. Indeed, without an organization behind you, it's almost impossible to get legislation passed to protect the rights of nonsmokers. A nonsmokers' rights group will give you clout, expertise, a central depot for information and activities, moral support, and some financial resources to battle the tobacco interests that will creep out of the woodwork once you announce you're seeking laws to protect nonsmokers. But the moral support is the most important thing. With a nonsmokers' rights group you'll know that you're not alone; you'll discover dozens of other people who feel the same way about tobacco smoke. Nonsmokers are the true silent majority (except when we cough because of cigarette fumes). Unlike the silent majority of the Nixon era, nonsmokers outnumber smokers three to one, and 86 percent of nonsmokers believe that smokers should refrain from lighting up in the presence of nonsmokers. Seventy-seven percent of *all* adults support workplace smoking restrictions—you're going to make some fast friends through your nonsmokers' rights group. Nonsmokers' rights groups around the country are connected in an informal network, so you'll be able to find out how other groups succeeded in passing nonsmokers' rights laws. These groups are usually called GASP (which stands for Group Against Smoking Pollution, or Group to Alleviate Smoking in Public). They frequently work in conjunction with the American Heart Association, American Lung Association, American Cancer Society, Action on Smoking and Health, and Americans for Nonsmokers' Rights.

The first step in starting your own GASP is the most difficult, but you've already taken it—deciding to form a nonsmokers' rights group. The Toledo, Ohio, GASP was founded by Patti H. Foley with friends she met in her allergist's office. Foley had to quit her job at a radio advertising company because exposure to smoke in clients' offices made her ill.[1] Ilene Freed was at a meeting of the local Lung Association where somebody asked, "Who wants to take over the nonsmokers' rights work?" She raised her hand and the next thing Ilene knew, she was president of Washingtonians for Nonsmokers' Rights.

If you've bought this book and you are reading this chapter, you're probably fed up with cigarette smoke around you. No doubt there have been more times than you can remember when your dinner out was rendered tasteless by a cigarette or two burning at the next table. Or you've been seated on an airplane in the so-called no-smoking section, three rows from where the smoking section begins and it's like going to an R. J. Reynolds board meeting. Or you'd like to find a no-smoking area in which to sit while you're waiting to board the plane. And you wonder how much sense it makes to allow smoking in hospital waiting rooms. You've tried to concentrate at work but the cigarette smoke wafting through the office has given you a headache, burning eyes, a cough—or all these ailments. And smoke-filled meetings are even worse. You notice that the clothing you wear to work or out to dinner smells like cigarettes afterward. You feel awkward about asking people at the next table in a restaurant not to smoke—and you don't because you're too polite or shy. Perhaps you're pregnant or have a small child with you and you're worried about the health of your offspring. You can't believe that smoking is allowed around small children and pregnant women, what with all the concern there is for the health of children. That's what annoys you most: There's all this scientific evidence that involuntary smoking is dangerous—it kills nonsmokers—and yet you can't escape it. All you want is to breathe safe, clean air.

You wonder, why are things often so backward? Shouldn't the presumption be pro-health—no smoking—instead of pro-disease?

Fortunately, the norm is changing in favor of common sense. And it's people like yourself who are changing things.

Most nonsmokers' rights organizations have several objectives:

- Enacting state or local workplace smoking restrictions.
- Enacting laws prohibiting smoking in all public places.
- Educating people about smoking and health.
- Providing consulting services to companies that want their own workplace smoking restrictions (private businesses are allowed to implement more restrictive regulations on smoking than specified in state or local laws).
- Learning about and developing strategies for asking people not to smoke.
- Working for national legislation to protect nonsmokers.
- Helping people use the law to protect themselves from cigarette smoke in the workplace and on airplanes.
- Getting media attention for nonsmokers' rights to help counter the cigarette companies' $2 billion-a-year advertising budget.

- Letting the tobacco industry know that the little guy can't be pushed around.
- Offering comradeship among nonsmokers.

Gather Information on Nonsmokers' Rights

The next step is to get some information about what other GASPs are doing. You should become educated and articulate on passive smoking. This book contains just about everything you need to know about involuntary smoking, but in addition, there are some organizations that can provide you with up-to-date or detailed material. Contact some of the nonsmokers' rights groups listed in Appendix A; tell them that you're starting a GASP group of your own and ask them for a copy of their newsletter and other information. Write and join Action on Smoking and Health and Americans for Nonsmokers Rights, and ask them for their current material on passive smoking. It's a good idea also to contact either the local or national chapters of the American Lung Association, American Heart Association, and American Cancer Society. Remember that these organizations depend on contributions for their work (unlike the cigarette companies), so a donation along with your request for information will go a long way toward supporting nonsmokers' rights.

Most groups are involved in innovative activities, so it won't be difficult to find out what's happening in the nonsmokers' rights movement around the country. Hawaii's nonsmokers' rights group, the Hawaiian Clean Air Team, has attracted attention by redefining "nonsmokers," calling them "clean air advocates." Instead of no-smoking sections, they are calling those spaces "clear air sections." (The converse is a "dirty air section.") Bowie GASP, in Maryland, keeps track of no-smoking retail establishments, and has even found a no-smoking beauty salon.

Action on Smoking and Health (ASH) has a myriad of nonsmokers' rights programs, which now includes Valentines for smokers.

Decide on a Name

It's a little thing, but having a name for your organization is a lot better than calling it "people concerned about smoking and health in our state.'' You can, of course, call your group Bridgton GASP or Tennessee GASP. Alternatives are Portlanders for Nonsmokers' Rights and Brooklynites Concerned About Smoking and Health. You should decide what region you want to focus on. If there's no state-wide nonsmokers' group in your state and you live in a major city, you might want to become the central group for your state. Or you might want to aim your efforts toward nonsmokers' rights in your town or county. It's fine to start small and expand as you acquire more members and money. Be sure to get in touch with the other nonsmokers' groups in your state and let them know about your plans so you can coordinate your activities and multiply your groups' influence.

Get Some Members

The tobacco companies and their allies aren't going to roll over and play dead or suddenly become dispassionate on issues that are vital to their survival, so you have a lot of work ahead of you. For every person you get on board your group, the easier it will be to achieve your objectives. Start with friends, coworkers, your physician, your aerobics instructor, people you see wheezing around cigarettes, and relatives. Ask them if they're bothered by cigarette smoke, tell them how it damages their health, and ask if they want to get involved. Talking with acquaintances is a start, but more than likely you'll need to go to other sources to find members.

Most of your membership-raising will progress slowly as people hear about your group through the media and by seeing your activities firsthand. People will want to join when they know exactly what you're doing and exactly how they can help.

Find out if there are any groups in your area that help people to quit smoking. Former smokers are frequently adamant nonsmokers' rights supporters because when they're around tobacco smoke they are tempted to reignite their habit.

The Basics

An address, phone number, stationery, bank account, and a brochure or fact sheet. These are the basics you need to get started. Although these initial expenses will have to come out of your pocket—or out of the pockets of your friends—your GASP can reimburse you later.

A post-office box is fine for your address, and an answering service or a separate phone line monitored by an answering machine will work for your phone number. The purpose of getting a P.O. box and a separate phone number is to make it easy for people to get in touch with you and to separate your professional and personal life from your smokers' rights activities. You'll need a bank account so that you can deposit checks written to your GASP group. The brochure doesn't need to be fancy; a simple message about cigarette smoking and your organization will be sufficient. (Always edit and proofread carefully!) Below is a sample brochure.

SAMPLE BROCHURE

Is Their Smoke Getting in Your Eyes?

If you're bothered by other people's cigarette smoke, now there's something you can do about it! Bethel GASP (Group Against Smoking Pollution) is fighting to protect your rights to breathe clean air at work, restaurants, and all public places.

For too long, nonsmokers have suffered when smokers were around. We've had to spend all day at work inhaling tobacco smoke, have had to endure meetings with almost unbreathable air, have had our meals at restaurants ruined by smoke at the table next to us, have had our clothes smell like stale cigarettes, and have worried about our health and the health of our children every time someone lights up around us.

Nonsmokers are tired of smoking other people's cigarettes!

We choose not to become involuntary smokers!

How Does Smoking Harm Nonsmokers?

And nonsmokers have every right to be concerned about involuntary cigarette smoking.

- A 1982 study by James Replace of the Environmental Protection Agency estimates that between five hundred and five thousand nonsmokers die each year of *lung cancer* from breathing sidestream cigarette smoke.
- J.R. White and H.F. Froeb reported in the *New England Journal of Medicine* that nonsmokers exposed to cigarette smoke in the workplace lost between 15 to 20 percent of their lung capacity.
- A study published in 1981 by T. Hirayama in the *British Medical Journal* found that nonsmoking wives of husbands who smoked heavily had almost twice the lung cancer rate of nonsmokers.
- Another study in the *American Journal of Epidemiology* in 1985 found that nonsmokers married to smokers had 60 percent more cancers of all kinds than people married to nonsmokers.
- The National Academy of Sciences said, "The Committee concludes that there is a positive association between lung cancer and chronic exposure to environmental tobacco smoke."
- Many nonsmokers experience coughing (25 percent) and headaches and nausea (30 percent) when exposed to cigarette smoke. According to one study, 70 percent of nonsmokers suffer eye irritation from cigarette smoke.
- Passive smoking causes abnormalities in the small airways of the lungs which may be a precursor to chronic lung disease, including emphysema.
- According to the Surgeon General's 1984 report, "The children of smoking parents have an increased prevalence of reported respiratory symptoms and have an increased frequency of bronchitis and pneumonia early in life."
- The Surgeon General said in 1982, "Sidestream smoke [contains] known carcinogens, some of which are in higher concentrations in sidestream smoke than they are in mainstream smoke."
- About twenty-five airplane fires are started by cigarettes or matches each year.
- The National Research Council has called for a ban on smoking on all airplanes, "to lessen irritation and discomfort to passengers and crew, to reduce potential health hazards to cabin crew . . . and to bring the cabin air quality into line with established standards for other closed environments."

What's so dangerous in sidestream smoke? Cigarette smoke contains over four thousand compounds. Some of the more notorious:

Dimethylnitrosamine (DMNA) is one of the most powerful cancer-causing substances known. According to *Chronic Diseases in Canada,* DMNA produces cancer in all animal species in which it has been tested and does so by various exposure routes including inhalation and after single doses.

Benzo(a)pyrene is another potent carcinogen in sidestream smoke.

Carbon monoxide, a colorless, odorless gas, has such a strong affinity for red blood cells that it successfully competes with oxygen for these cells. As the amount of the molecule increases in your blood, your body is deprived of oxygen. The average CO level next to a smoker is ninety parts per million—nearly twice the level considered safe for industrial exposure. *Nitrogen dioxide* and *hydrogen cyanide* are two other dangerous gasses found in sidestream smoke.

Nicotine makes the heart beat faster (while carbon dioxide is robbing the blood of oxygen).

Polonium-210 is a *radioactive* element associated with cancer.

Sidestream smoke also contains *ammonia, formaldehyde,* and *arsenic.*

Ventilation Usually Can't Clean the Air

Most office buildings recirculate their air, rather than infusing the building with fresh air. Only 10 percent fresh air is added to indoor air each hour, so as the day progresses, the building's atmosphere becomes more and more polluted. Most of the dangerous substances in tobacco smoke are odorless, tasteless, and invisible.

In restaurants and airplanes ventilation isn't any better. As Dick Cavett said, "Anyone with half a brain knows that to refer to the no-smoking section of a plane is like saying the no-chlorine section of the pool."

Most Americans Want Restrictions on Smoking in Public

Bethel GASP is part of one of the largest majorities in the country. A 1987 Gallup poll showed that 76 percent of former smokers, and 64 percent of current smokers believe that smokers should refrain from lighting up in the presence of nonsmokers. In answer to the question, "Should companies have a policy on smoking at work?" 92 percent of nonsmokers, 80 percent of smokers, and 89 percent of former smokers said YES!

The popularity of no smoking can be measured in nonquantitative ways, too. On a packed TWA flight between St. Louis and Los Angeles everyone in the smoking section was smoking, and the air in that section was so thick from tobacco fumes that flight attendants drew straws to see who would have to work in that section. Later in the flight the entire plane became saturated with cigarette smoke—even the rest rooms. Passengers traveling in coach were permitted to use the lavatories in the first class section. Finally when the captain switched on the no-smoking sign, some passengers applauded.[2]

But What About the "Rights" of Smokers?

Smoking is not a right, it's a limited privilege. People's so-called right to smoke ends where our lungs begin; nobody has the right to pursue an activity that harms others. But being able to breathe clean air is a right and that's what Bethel GASP is fighting for.

"Common courtesy"—the slogan of the tobacco companies—isn't the answer. Nonsmokers shouldn't be constantly put in the awkward position of asking every time someone lights up, "Excuse me, would you mind not smoking?" It's tiresome, embarrassing, and let's face it, sometimes stressful. Besides, smokers aren't always reasonable about their behavior, as you would expect from a habit that's physically and psychologically addictive. If common courtesy were the answer, then smokers would automatically *not* light up around nonsmokers (especially children and pregnant women).

Fortunately, the majority of both nonsmokers and smokers prefer laws on smoking in public places. In addition to protecting health, nonsmokers' rights laws are the best way to prevent disputes between smokers and nonsmokers. These laws promote courtesy!

Smoking in the Workplace Is Also Expensive

Workplace smoking restrictions reduce costs for businesses.

- Each smoker costs his employer $350 a year in short-term expenses such as increased cleaning, furniture and equipment maintenance, fire, health and life insurance premiums, and lost productivity, and $1,000 a year in long-term costs such as premature disability and death.

- Each nonsmoker exposed to passive smoke at the workplace costs her employer $50 a year in short-term costs and $100 every year in long-term costs.
- Workers at Dow Chemical's Midland, Texas, plant were absent 5.5 days a year more than nonsmokers, costing the company $657,146 in excess wage costs alone.
- Pacific Northwest Bell discovered that the lifetime cost of smoking for a forty-year-old who smokes two packs a day is $56,670.
- Johnson & Johnson has cut absenteeism by 20 percent and hospitalizations by 30 percent through its workplace smoking policies and by helping smokers quit. The savings have been three times the cost of implementing these programs.

Nonsmokers pay a heavy price for other people's smoking habits—not only in terms of health, but through our pocketbooks, too.

What Is Bethel GASP?

Bethel GASP is working for:

- Smokefree workplaces.
- Separate smoking and no-smoking sections in restaurants.
- No smoking in public places including transportation, health-care facilities, day-care centers, public meeting rooms.
- Federal laws to protect nonsmokers.
- A ban on smoking on airplanes.
- Restricting smoking in the waiting lounges at the Bethel airport and train station.
- Education of more people about smoking, involuntary smoking, and health.

We're going to be facing a tough battle. The tobacco industry is a $40-billion-a-year business; cigarette companies dispense over $2 billion *a year* on advertising; the Tobacco Institute and its allies spend hundreds of thousands or more dollars when there's a legislative campaign to ban smoking. We expect to be outspent. We expect that the people of Bethel will be lied to. ("What many of us haven't recognized is the consistent failure of scientists to establish any ingredient—or group of ingredients—

in the quantity found in tobacco smoke as the cause of any human disease" reads one Tobacco Institute publication.)

But we expect to win. Because over the past five years nonsmokers' rights groups around the country have achieved remarkable success in enacting nonsmokers' rights laws. In places like Cambridge, Massachusetts, Fairfax, Virginia, Berkeley, California, and New York City.

And soon in Bethel, Maine.

Join Bethel GASP. Membership is only fifteen dollars a year, a small price for healthy lungs. Feel free to write or call us for more information.

Bethel GASP
P.O. Box 12345
Bethel, Maine 12345
207-555-6789

Pass the brochure around. Give copies to your coworkers, maybe even distribute some on a street corner. Slip copies under cars' windshield wipers at hospital parking lots. Post copies on bulletin boards in your local markets and on kiosks. Ask store managers if they'll allow you to put a flier in their window or perhaps leave a pile for people to pick up inside. Make the same request at your local hospital. Distribute leaflets wherever and whenever possible.

Action on Smoking and Health, the foremost smoking and health organization in the country, will provide your organization with a list of ASH's members for a mailing. ASH's address is listed in Appendix A. ASH can be helpful in innumerable ways—it has more experience battling cigarette companies than any other organization. Anne Morrow Donley, president of Virginia GASP, says, "Exchanging newsletters and information is vital. That's where ASH has been so great. I can't sing their praises enough. They sent us stickers for the press booklets . . . when I made a desperate call to rush them (after being struck with the brilliant idea to have them)."

Form a Steering Committee

The Steering Committee is going to be the workhorse of your nonsmokers' rights organization. They're the people who will make most of the decisions for the organization and do most of the work. It's a good idea to have some notables on your steering committee who may be less active, but can lend prestige to your group. Doctors are a good place to start, because there's not a physician in America who thinks smoking is good for you. Ask your local heart, lung, and cancer associations and any environmental groups if they can lend some of their officials to be on your steering committee; chances are that they will want to. Your local fire station is also a good source of members for your core group, because smoking causes a large percent of all residential fires. Call some businesses in the area to see if they have workplace smoking restrictions; nonsmoking employees of companies that do are often keenly interested in supporting restrictions on smoking in public places, too. Find out if any restaurants around town or in the state have no-smoking sections, and ask their owners to participate.

You should be well on your way toward building a solid and effective nonsmokers' rights organization.

Attracting More Members and More Funds

Anyone who has a mailbox already knows the most effective fundraising and membership gathering tool—direct mail. Some of the most successful letters come not from national organizations, but from local groups, like yours. So a mailing should be one of your first activities.

The mechanics of a direct mailing aren't complicated, but there are a lot of details involved such as obtaining a bulk mailing permit (or not), using business reply envelopes (or not), determining exactly how much money to ask for (give recipients choices, and give them large choices), deciding what to put on the outside of the envelope (getting people to open the envelope is the most important component of any direct-mail campaign), which mailing lists to use (the heart, lung, cancer, and other groups in your area may lend you their names for a mailing), whether to use individualized letters (or a form letter), and so forth. There are a lot of good books available on selling through direct mail, and there are a lot of good consultants on direct-mail marketing. It's worthwhile getting one or the other.

You'll discover that nonsmokers are a diverse group. According to Anne Morrow Donley, ''Nonsmokers are drawn from all walks of life and various political persuasions, and may not necessarily agree on other topics. This is important to remember.'' Indeed, even smokers may join your organization. Don't talk about Nicaragua or abortion in your GASP: Focus on involuntary smoking.

Treating your membership properly is vital, too. People join non-smokers' rights organizations because they are concerned and want to become involved. Donley says it's ''very important . . . to make certain that everyone feels a part of the group. I've tried extra hard to make certain everyone has a say. I send out memos to the active members, giving ideas and urging their feedback. And they give it. Sometimes it's just, 'okay, do it'; sometimes it's highly critical and constructive; sometimes we end up brainstorming into something quite different.''

Donley adds another thought: ''Don't expect crowds at your meetings. Expect maybe five to ten people at most.'' You should never use the size of your meetings as a barometer for how effective your organization will be. In fact, a tremendous amount can be accomplished with just a handful of volunteers.

Raising Money

While memberships and solicitations through the mail will bring in some capital, and you will have a lot of volunteer support (in contrast to the tobacco industry which pays everyone who helps them very hefty salaries), it's still true that in political activity the more money you have the more you will be able to accomplish.

Always thank your contributors with a letter or phone call. This is the most crucial rule of fundraising. Every donor wants to believe that her contribution is making a difference.

Apply with the Internal Revenue Service for tax-exempt or tax-deductible status.

A newsletter is a must for any nonsmokers' rights organization. Through your newsletter you can keep members informed about your group's activities, about what other GASPs are doing, what the cancer, heart, and lung associations are up to, and what's happening in Congress, *how and whom to lobby on nonsmokers' rights legislation pending in your state legislature,* companies that have instituted workplace smoking restrictions, new research about passive smoking, recent Tobacco Institute distortions, ideas on how to ask smokers how to stop, and ways to contribute more to your organization. You might also include the names of local legislators who received the most money from the Tobacco Institute. The newsletter does not have to appear frequently—monthly, quarterly, or even twice a year is okay, but it must be published on a schedule. Try soliciting advertisements from restaurants that have no-smoking sections, insurance companies that offer reduced policies to nonsmokers (and insurance agents), health food stores, and medical groups. You'll find that these advertisements will cover the cost of your newsletter.

Membership cards are inexpensive and make members feel welcome. They will help with contributions.

Selling is always an effective tool for fundraising. People are more willing donors when they receive something tangible. T-shirts are a good way of raising money (they can say something like "No-Smoking Section"), as are buttons, bumper stickers, and No-Smoking signs. You can borrow an idea from the D.C. Lung Association and sell stickers that say "I enjoyed dining here, but wish you had a Nonsmoking Section," along with your group's name and phone number.

Media

The press is extremely important to your group. A good story in the paper or on TV or radio news may do more for your association and for enacting laws to protect nonsmokers than any amount of brochures. Politicians pay attention to the news and often use local press coverage as a measure of public opinion. Compile a list of newspapers, magazines, radio, and television stations in your areas. When you send press releases to these organizations, address the releases to the particular reporters who cover issues related to nonsmokers' rights— notices sent to the City Desk often wind up in the city garbage can. It's fine to send press releases to more than one person on a paper.

Get in touch with the hosts of talk shows on your local radio and television stations. They're always looking for new, interesting guests—some love controversy. When there's a new report about tobacco and health, or when the cigarette companies release their annual reports, volunteer to speak on behalf of the 75 percent of Americans who do not smoke.

Here's a sample letter you can send to radio stations, patterned after a letter used by Washingtonians for Nonsmokers' Rights:

Dear Radio Host:

One of the most controversial—and important—issues in the Washington area is cigarette smoking in public. During the next year the District of Columbia City Council and local governments in Maryland and Virginia are expected to vote on legislation prohibiting smoking in the workplace, restaurants, and other public places.

Ilene Freed, president of Washingtonians for Nonsmokers Rights, is available for interviews in your studio and by phone. Washingtonians for Nonsmokers' Rights was formed last year by Ms. Freed to promote legislation and business practices that prohibit tobacco smoking.

"Most people understand that tobacco is bad for smokers," Ms. Freed said. "But what many don't recognize is that secondhand or involuntary cigarette smoke can be deadly. There is now ample evidence showing that thousands of Americans may be dying each year from involuntary cigarette smoke."

Smoking is the most significant public health problem in America. More Americans—about 350,000 each year—die from cigarettes than are killed by alcohol, cocaine, heroin, PCP, and all other drugs combined. Yet cigarettes are the most heavily advertised product in the world—cigarette companies spend over $2 billion a year pushing their products.

Restrictions on smoking in the workplace, restaurants, and other public locations have worked virtually perfectly in San Francisco, East Lansing, Michigan, San Diego—everywhere nonsmokers' rights legislation has passed. Prohibiting smoking in public places has not only improved public health, but has saved money. Cleaning costs in restaurants and absentee rates in businesses drop when smoking is not allowed.

"People have a right to breathe clean air," Ms. Freed pointed out. "Our objective is as simple as that.

"We expect Washington, D.C., to be a major battle ground for nonsmokers' rights legislation," said Freed. "After all, this is the nation's capital and the Tobacco Institute is housed here. The tobacco companies cannot afford to see nonsmokers' rights legislation pass in Washington." She added, "Despite over fifty thousand studies pointing to the dangers of cigarettes,

you'll never get a spokesperson to admit that cigarette smoking
is unhealthy.''

To arrange an interview with Ilene Freed, please call (202)
555-1990.

Generally, you have to tie your media efforts to your group's
activities. Reporters are more receptive to writing about a subject when
there's something newsworthy.

Organizing a Press Conference

When you have something that's particularly newsworthy to announce, or are organizing an unusual event, call a press conference. A
press conference gives reporters an opportunity to meet your group's
leaders, to ask questions, and to probe deeply into GASP's plans and
motives.

A press conference is only successful if the press comes. Press
conferences can be a little like false alarms, too: You can get away
with calling one that isn't newsworthy—once; after that the press
won't show up. So give reporters a reason to attend. Reporters gather
at press conferences if one of three conditions are met. First, if your
activity involves a lot of people, that's news. There's little worse for
a newspaper than dozens of individuals writing to the paper, asking,
"Why didn't you cover this event?" Second, reporters like to attend
press conferences that offer views counter to those enunciated by other
organizations. For example, in 1986 Virginia GASP organized a press
conference on passive smoking and health in the same Richmond,
Virginia building at which the annual Tobacco Expo was being held.
Doing that took a lot of chutzpah, and the press conference received a
commensurate amount of attention. Third, if you have something
especially newsworthy to announce, the press will attend. For example,
if you're announcing the introduction of legislation to ban smoking in
public places or you have evidence that the cigarette companies from
outside the state are spending hundreds of thousands of dollars against
the effort to pass a law regulating smoking in buildings, that's news.

Press conferences should be interesting. Reporters are regular
people, too, and tire quickly of the standard let's-announce-this-
and-pass-out-our-statement press conference. The look of the press

conference may be as important as what you say. John Banzhaf, ASH's founder, recommends having a visual press conference with smoking-related artifacts around the room. Groups which have followed his advice have received considerable attention. Put some antismoking posters on the wall. Run the films *Secondhand Smoke* or *Death in the West* silently while your press conference is underway. Alternatively, show the Department of Health and Human Services' don't-smoke-around-babies public service announcement. Get someone to dress as the Grim Reaper and just stand there the whole while. Prepare a three-dimensional bar graph with one side showing how much money the tobacco companies spend on advertising each year—made up of a stack of cigarette packs—versus how much money is spent in the U.S. warning people about the dangers of smoking—made up of a stack of pennies. Or put an ashtray with cigarette butts next to a rose in a clear vase, with a sign in front of both asking, "Which would you prefer to sit next to at work?" Give photographers something to take a picture of—it'll increase your chances of appearing on tonight's television news or in tomorrow's paper. Bundle your material into a press kit for reporters to take home; put your statement, press release, a brochure on passive smoking, a flier on the history of the nonsmokers' rights movement, buttons, a bumper sticker, and even a prepared photograph of your display into a folder with pockets.

Consider timing your press conference to another tobacco-related event such as the Great American Smokeout, sponsored by the American Cancer Society each November, or the release of the Surgeon General's annual report on smoking and health. Alternatively, schedule your press conference on the day that Philip Morris or R.J. Reynolds releases their annual reports. The press will already be covering these events and will be looking for a local angle, as well. You can be that local angle.

Action

Action is what your group is all about. There's a wide range of activities you can pursue—more than you will have the funds or volunteers for—so you will have to decide which efforts should receive the most attention. What follows is a list of suggested activities.

- Informing people about the hazards of involuntary smoking and telling them how they can improve the quality of the air they breathe are among your most important tasks. Education should be a constant effort, because it is your most natural and vital ally. It should take many forms, including placing op-ed articles in your local papers. You should also keep the public abreast of the tobacco companies' activities and lies.

   Be prepared to counter tobacco industry tactics. Cigarette companies have shifted their strategies and are now aggressively pretending that the cigarette industry isn't treated well by the media. The tobacco industry is also focusing on smoking as a civil rights issue, rather than as a question of health. Don't let the Tobacco Institute frame the debate: Talk about the Surgeon General's report; mention the Replace-Lowrey study and the National Academy of Sciences' conclusions. Let the credibility of the cigarette companies become an issue: If they won't acknowledge that mainstream smoking is dangerous, they can't be believed about anything. Reveal the tobacco industry's biases and lies.

- A petition drive is a good way to let people know about your group. The petitions can ask citizens whether they support no smoking in public places, as well as separating smokers and nonsmokers at restaurants and at work. Or, more purposefully, you can launch a petition drive to get state legislators to introduce nonsmokers' rights laws. Legislative activities should be one of your group's primary objectives. Keep working at getting one of your state legislators or city council members to introduce a bill to protect nonsmokers (which, you should always remind them, includes children and fetuses). Once legislation is introduced it's always helpful to have average citizens call or write their representatives and express their feelings about laws protecting nonsmokers' rights. These sentiments should be simple and direct. GASP of Colorado recommends simply saying: "I heard on the radio (or TV) (or read in the newspaper) about this ordinance restricting smoking in public places. I think it is great, and I would like you to support it by voting in favor of it."

- Collect evidence about smoking and children and release it to the press. Call for no smoking in schools by anyone; propose legislation to prohibit cigarette vending machines, which are how most children buy their cigarettes. Probably the best vehicle for banning smoking in school is the school board. If the school has an antidrug program, try to get cigarettes to be part of that campaign. After all, in 1985, smoking killed a hundred times as many people as cocaine did.

- Work to pass local ordinances to ban cigarette advertising on the bus and subway lines on which children ride to school.
- One-up tobacco industry p.r. efforts. When Philip Morris announced a contest that awarded $15,000 to the best essay about freedom of the press (which *Cincinnati Enquirer* columnist Tony Lang dubbed the "Buy-A-Journalist Contest"), the antismoking group, Doctors Ought to Care (DOC), headed by Dr. Alan Blum, had a better idea. Cosponsored with the Tobacco Products Liability Project, the DOC contest awarded $1,000 to the best essay on the question: "Are tobacco company executives responsible for the deaths, diseases, and fires their products cause?"
- Many GASPs are actively protesting the Virginia Slims Tennis Tournament by holding an *Emphysema Slims* press conference the day of the tournament. In 1986, Virginia GASP, Northern Virginia GASP, and Washingtonians for Nonsmokers' Rights picketed the tournaments to alert people to the incongruity of a cigarette company sponsoring an athletic event. These groups wanted to make clear their belief that Philip Morris shouldn't be allowed to use tennis tournaments to accumulate goodwill and promote the notion that cigarettes are indeed an element of sports. Cigarette companies are fond of sponsoring athletic competitions, because they bolster the *feeling* that cigarettes are safe. Philip Morris required tennis tournament ball boys and girls to wear Virginia Slims T-shirts depicting a woman holding a cigarette. Mary Elliot Kozak, head of Northern Virginia GASP, called these boys and girls "walking tobacco billboards."
- Activate local retailers. Safeway food stores responded to complaints from nonsmokers by posting signs in their stores around the country that proclaim: "Thank You for Not Smoking in a Food Store."

- Publish a list of restaurants and other places that have separate smoking and no-smoking sections. Encourage people to patronize these establishments. Let restaurants know that if they provide a no-smoking section you'll give them free mentions in your newsletter.
- Get local hotels involved. Hotels are gradually recognizing that no smoking means good business, according to *The Wall Street Journal,* which reported that most major hotel firms provide at least 5 percent of their rooms for nonsmokers.[3] Said Gerald Petitt, executive vice president of Quality Inns International, ''About 65 percent of the population is interested in no-smoking accommodations, more than for any other hotel amenities, such as flowers or chocolates.'' Encourage hotels in your town to offer no-smoking rooms or floors; no smoking saves hotels money through reduced cleaning and furniture replacement costs. Quality Inns discovered that smokeless rooms cost 26 percent less to clean. And remember, tobacco smoke flows through a hotel's ventilation system, contaminating rooms throughout the building.
- Hand out literature on smoking and health whenever cigarette samples or discount coupons for cigarettes are given away.
- Contact your local public and commercial television stations and encourage them to broadcast a documentary about cigarette smoking. Some public television stations may be interested in preparing their own, but there are a few good documentaries available for rent. One, which has an interesting history, is called *Death in the West,* a 1976 British film produced by Thames Television, that traces the lives of the five original Marlboro men—real, American cowboys—who appeared in Philip Morris's TV commercials. This chilling documentary also contains interviews with executives of Philip Morris, and contrasts the rugged Marlboro image with the fate of these five cowboys: lung surgery, oxygen tanks, cobalt radiation treatment—agony. Four died of either lung cancer or emphysema. Soon after the film was broadcast in England, Philip Morris obtained an injunction banning the film from being seen in the United States. Even

60 Minutes was unable to broadcast it! Then, five years later, Dr. Stanton Glantz of the University of California Medical School, received an unsolicited package containing *Death in the West*. The following year *Death in the West* was shown around the country—despite the legal dangers. Copies of *Death in the West* can be obtained from Americans for Nonsmokers' Rights. *Secondhand Smoke* is another excellent documentary that's available from Pyramid films.

- Offer materials and guidance to local firms. Eventually you will have developed enough expertise on passive smoking to either publish a booklet for companies that want to have workplace smoking restrictions, or provide consulting services on how to implement no-smoking policies.

- Be present at tobacco-sponsored events, as Virginia GASP was at the 1986 Tobacco Expo. They were surrounded by manufacturers of cigarettes, cigarette papers, tobacco growers—and the media. Your group is bound to get noticed at such events.

- Airport waiting areas are good targets for nonsmokers' rights activities. If airplanes have no-smoking sections, doesn't it make sense that lounges in airports should be treated similarly? A better goal is to pursue no smoking at all at airports. Children, pregnant women, not to mention people with allergies and sensitivities to tobacco smoke, have to wait in airports with smokers; a minority of smokers are subjecting these people to harmful fumes and particles. It's unfair. Write the manager at your local airport and then start lobbying the state or city board that regulates the airport. If nothing else, they will be receptive to your argument that no smoking reduces cleaning costs. You can also have a physical presence at airports. Any group has the right to hand out material and solicit contributions at airports—you'll find that just after travelers have left a smoke-filled airplane they will be most receptive to your group's goals.

- Host nonsmoking parties, dances, and dinners. It's rare, almost impossible, to find anyplace to go out where there's no smoking. Try to convince a bar owner to have a no-smoking night as an experiment. Let musical performers who are coming to town know that they can request that the management prohibit smoking during the night they're on stage.

- Sponsor a turn-in-your-ashtray day. Everyone who turns in an ashtray will receive a 10 percent discount on dinner at one of several restaurants with clean-air dining.
- Demonstrate in front of events that are sponsored by tobacco companies, especially sporting events. Let people know that tobacco does not promote sports or health, even though sports is used to promote tobacco.
- Get the doctors in town to become members of your organization. Prepare a special pamphlet that physicians can distribute to their patients about smoking, passive smoking, and smoking and children.
- If there are any singers on your team, we'll be happy to send complimentary copies of the music to "Careless Smoker," the lyrics of which are given on pages 11 and 12.
- Design "Congratulations for Quitting" cards and sell them. You may find a couple of local stores that are willing to carry them. If there's an artist in your GASP, design an attractive *Thank You for Not Smoking* sign.
- Encourage cab companies to offer no-smoking cabs, to provide no-smoking cabs on request, or to mark taxis "No Smoking" on the outside.
- Make sure that local ordinances and other regulations on smoking are enforced. Many supermarkets, for example, have to have no smoking for insurance purposes, but this may not be enforced. Your group can be instrumental in helping workers ensure that their companies' workplace smoking restrictions are adhered to.
- The most radical action taken by a nonsmokers' rights organization was organized in Australia by a group called BUGAUP (Billboard Utilizing Graffitists Against Unhealthy Promotions). In the states of Western Australia, Tasmania, the Australian Capital Territory, and South Australia, antismokers used spray paint to modify billboards. A Dunhill advertisement became "Lung Ill"; a Benson & Hedges sign had the phrase, "Their Gold—Your Lungs" added to it; Rothmans King Size became "Rot Mans Lung

Size." Fred Cole, a spokesman for the group said, "The automatic reaction is that property is sacred. More so than people's lives. When you think about it and realize the harm they're doing, where does the morality lie?" Dr. Michael Lippman of Seattle, Washington, inspired by BUGAUP, was arrested in December 1985 for modifying a Camel Filters billboard. The original read "CAMEL FILTERS— It's a whole new world." Dr. Lippman added, "OF CANCER." He was arrested, of course, and charged with destruction of property. The doctor explained, "As a family doctor . . . I get people with severe emphysema, lung cancer, chronic bronchitis, heart disease. Why should we allow advertising for a substance that kills? My feeling is that cigarette smoking is a contagious disease, and that advertising is the carrier."

- Find nonsmokers' rights issues to fight for; it's not hard. Virginia GASP is spearheading an effort to get smokefree waiting areas in hospitals. When Dorothy Jones brought her husband to the waiting area in the emergency room at Waynesboro Community Hospital, she couldn't find any no-smoking area in which to sit. Even though she and her husband are acutely allergic to tobacco smoke, nobody in the hospital would bring them chairs so that they could sit near the door. Amazing—hospitals without clean-air sections. Virginia GASP recommends writing complaints to the Joint Commission on Accreditation of Health Care Organizations, 875 North Michigan Avenue, Chicago, IL 60611. Write your own state hospital association to request no-smoking sections in hospitals. Many of the same techniques used to get smokefree workplaces can be used to eliminate smoking in hospitals.

- Write literature that pokes fun at the cigarette companies. Satire and humor can be powerful tools in moving people to peer through the Tobacco Institute's propaganda; satire and its cousin ridicule can move people's intellect and emotions. What follows is an example of how poking fun at the cigarette industry can highlight the flaws in its arguments:

A PARODY
THE T.L.K. TOBACCO COMPANY ANSWERS SOME TOUGH QUESTIONS ABOUT SMOKING

Numerous studies appear to link cancer and smoking. Once and for all: Does cigarette smoking cause cancer?

No.

What about those studies?

The so-called evidence is merely circumstantial. No cause-and-effect relationship has ever been established between smoking and cancer. If a mouse gets cancer from being exposed to tremendous volumes of cigarette smoke, as they are in these tests, it does not mean that people will get cancer. After all, mice are chased by cats, but people and cats get along fine.

Besides, you have to take into account that these studies are funded by zealous antismoking groups, wealthy individuals who erroneously claim to have lost relatives because of supposed cancer-inducing cigarette smoking, and people who are too lazy to buy ash trays.

What evidence is there that smoking is safe?

A 1984 study performed by the Wheeler Clinic of North Carolina concluded that there is no link between cancer and tobacco. In 1982 the vice-president of the Cancer Association, no friend of cigarettes, said, "[S]moking . . . puts individuals at no . . . great . . . health risk . . ."

What about heart disease?

The average person breathes more harmful gasses, including carbon monoxide, standing in line to get on a city bus or tailgating a truck, than smoking hundreds of packs of cigarettes a day. In fact, independent studies show that one of the largest environmental causes of heart disease is putting on clothing just after they've come back from the drycleaners.

Aren't nonsmokers harmed by "secondhand" cigarette smoke?

No.

What can someone do who's sitting next to a smoker but is bothered by the smoke?

First, we suggest turning the other cheek. If a nonsmoker is continually bothered by another's cigarette smoke it's crucial that he seek professional psychiatric help.

Should smokers be segregated from nonsmokers in restaurants, offices, and airplanes?

That's not really a recipe for social harmony. It's bound to lead to further discord and the breaking apart of families in which only some members smoke. These families won't be able to eat, work, or fly together.

Segregation of smokers is as bad as any other kind of segregation. We ought not discriminate against the smoker. Instead, we should pursue the only alternative—fairness. We should seek peaceful coexistence, civility, and sensibility.

Aren't smokers inconsiderate by not asking whether the person sitting next to them minds before lighting up?

We encourage smokers and nonsmokers to engage in a reasonable, adult dialogue about smoking. But there would be no such dialogue if smokers never lit up. That's why the tobacco companies are here: to promote harmony and happiness. We've made great progress since the first peace pipes were passed between Indians and European settlers. We want to continue that record.

Why smoke?

Smoking is a personal decision, like having sex. People smoke because lighting up gives them pleasure. Fortunately, Americans are blessed with hundreds of cigarette brands from which to choose.

Should minors smoke?

Smoking is an adult custom. Adults enjoy smoking because we need a calming, satisfying, and flavorful habit. Children have their own habits. So, we guess the answer to your question is that children shouldn't be encouraged to smoke. And you'll notice that our advertisements are specifically designed not to appeal to minors.

Are warnings on cigarette packages resasonable?

Absolutely not. First, cigarettes are safe, so the warnings aren't necessary. Second, the cost of printing these messages is passed along to the customer, resulting in higher cigarette prices and less disposable income for consumers. The consequence is a less vigorous economy. Historically speaking, we had more employment, less inflation, and a smaller deficit before these messages were required. There is a strong link between government-induced messages and a weak American economy.

What about litter? I'm always seeing discarded cigarettes along the sidewalk and road.

If there were no cigarettes, smokers would find other objects to litter with, such as paper clips and gum wrappers. The amount of litter generated would be the same.

The government wants cigarette companies to list the ingredients in their product. What are the implications of this?

It would be a step backward in the effort to promote civil liberties. Once tobacco companies are forced to reveal what makes their cigarettes special, there will be no stopping government intrusion into our private lives.

The T.L.K. Tobacco Company is spending a lot of money on these advertisements. Why?

We want people to know the truth.

Brought to you in the public interest
from your friends at
T.L.K. (Tough Luck Kiddo) Tobacco

Get Involved in Congressional Legislation

Although the primary purpose of your nonsmokers' rights group is to advance legislation in your community to protect the air that smokers and nonsmokers breathe, Congress has often been a prime mover in nonsmokers' rights statutes. One key area is airlines. In 1988 Congress passed legislation prohibiting smoking on all domestic flights of less than two hours, affecting 80 percent of all passengers. Only 12 percent of airline passengers want to sit in smoking sections. This legislation was the first step—and a major step—toward getting a total ban on all domestic flights. But the ban still is an experiment, and it expires in 1990. So if we are to get a total smoking ban on domestic flights, it will be only because of your efforts.

Tobacco smoke on airlines, by the way, flows quite freely into the cockpit. This may affect the safety of aircraft, according to Captain H.B. Fulton, Jr. In his prepared testimony to Congress, Captain Fulton reported:

One of the numerous byproducts of smoking is tobacco tar, a sticky brownish-black substance that can wreak havoc with sensitive aircraft systems. The pressurization is controlled by the outflow valve which becomes gummed up and functions erratically or not at all and can cause pressurization malfunctions. Instruments and computers utilize cockpit and cabin air for cooling and the filters and mechanisms in these systems become contaminated much sooner with air containing tobacco smoke . . . In a survey by the Air Line Pilots Association to 1,287 pilots, 80 percent of the respondents reported 23 detrimental physical reactions including eye irritation, headache, difficulty breathing, nose/sinus irritation, and increased fatigue.[4]

Does anybody out there want pilots in less-than-perfect shape for flying?

There's another way to look at smoking on airlines, too: "The lighting of small fires onboard an airliner high in the sky is idiotic," said Captain Fulton.

When burned, the materials in the cabin and seats give off an extremely dense and toxic smoke. Once a fire is established the only procedure available to the crew is to fight the fire with hand-held extinguishers. If, as in the case of some of the lavatory fires the industry has experienced, the fire has time to penetrate the interior skin of the fuselage, a hand-held extinguisher is nearly useless. . . . There is nothing that can be done now except land as soon as possible and hope that you have not suffocated in the meantime.[5]

Is an in-flight fire likely? Several have started in rest rooms. So many lit cigarettes are dropped on flights that attendants don't bother to report them. At least one aircraft, an Air Canada DC-9, is thought to have burned because a cigarette was tossed in the paper disposal in the rest room.

Congress is active on a number of other fronts: In 1987, a provision to a spending bill was added that would have cut $539 million in assistance to New York's Metropolitan Transportation Authority unless smoking was banned on the Long Island Rail Road. Guess what? Smoking was banned on the L.I.R.R. quite promptly. (According to the railroad, only 12 percent of its passengers wanted to sit in smoking cars, even though 37 percent smoked.)

In 1988 Senator Bill Bradley (D–New Jersey) introduced a bill requiring a label be placed on all tobacco products and advertising: "Warning: Smoking is addictive. Once you start you may not be able to stop.'' Senator Bradley, along with Congressman Fortney H. (Pete) Stark (D–California) have proposed repealing legislation that obstructs tobacco product-liability lawsuits. Every few years legislation is introduced to raise the tax on cigarettes. (The current federal tax is sixteen cents a pack. States may also charge tax on cigarettes, and this issue comes before state legislatures as well.) When the tax goes up, fewer people smoke, and fewer teenagers start smoking. The net result of higher cigarette taxes is less passive smoke all around. These are all important issues for nonsmokers' rights groups.

Other strong antismoking legislation that could have an impact on nonsmokers' rights has been considered by Congress. In 1987 Representatives Bob Whittaker (R–Kansas) and Jim Bates (D–California) introduced legislation calling for tobacco products to be brought under the jurisdiction of the Food and Drug Administration (FDA). The bill, the Comprehensive Tobacco Health and Safety Act, would have also required that cigarette companies add a label warning of tobacco addictiveness, list all additives, and ban the sale of tobacco to people under eighteen years old. Additives are a particularly curious thing: Nobody besides the tobacco companies knows what goes into cigarettes. In fact, most of the tobacco companies' testing of additives goes on overseas. Why overseas? In the event that an additive is found to be dangerous, it would be very difficult for American courts to discover the results of those tests.[6]

Remember that Congress is not totally pro-nonsmokers' rights. Otherwise there would be a total ban on smoking on airlines, federal protection against cigarette smoke in public places and the workplace, no cigarette vending machines (where minors buy most of their cigarettes), and even stronger warnings on cigarette packages. Tobacco states elect pro-tobacco representatives and senators; these members of Congress trade for pro-cigarette votes with members from nontobacco-producing states. The tobacco industry is a major contributor to congressional campaigns and is the fourth highest payer of speaking fees to members of Congress—$135,000 in 1985.

There's plenty for your nonsmokers' rights group to do.

NOTES

(1) *Cleveland Plain Dealer,* April 6, 1986, p. P31.
(2) *Los Angeles Times,* March 30, 1986, part 7, p. 2.
(3) *The Wall Street Journal,* December 4, 1986, p. 37.
(4) Captain H.B. Fulton, Jr., "Hearing on Legislation to Ban Smoking on Airline Aircraft," U.S. House of Representatives, Subcommittee on Aviation, October 7, 1987.
(5) *Ibid.*
(6) John Slade, M.D., *New Jersey Medicine,* February 1988, p. 105.

CHAPTER 4

Enacting Nonsmokers' Rights Laws Part I: The Legislation

SMOKING: A custome lothsome to the Eye, hateful to the Nose, harmful to the Braine, dangerous to the Lungs, and, in the black stinking Fume thereof, nearest resembling the horrible Stygian Smoke of the Pit that is bottomless.

King James I of England, 1604

Enacting legislation to protect the health of smokers in public places may be the most important role of any nonsmokers' rights organization. Nonsmokers' rights groups around the country are vigorously pursuing laws to prohibit or restrict smoking in public places such as restaurants, elevators, workplaces, public transportation, taxis, waiting rooms, concert halls, movie theaters, hospitals (yes, many hospitals allow smoking inside), convention centers—everywhere the public gathers. Passing legislation is a formidable task, one that is not made easier by the fact that the tobacco lobby is 100 percent and millions of dollars against it. But groups which have embarked on this course have been successful in realizing their goal, not necessarily on the first try, but eventually. And, just as important, once enacted, laws restricting smoking in public places have been completely effective, troublefree and permanent.

The key to passing legislation on the state or local level is *influence*, the essential ingredient of politics everywhere in the world. Influence comes in a variety of colors: money, prestige, who you know, popular appeal, press appeal, timing, persistence, good luck, and moral suasion. Your GASP will have to employ a mix of all these elements in order for nonsmokers' rights to spread to your area. But that's not too difficult to do, because the concept of nonsmokers' rights legislation is so powerful that the colors of influence will naturally drift toward you.

Nonsmokers' rights legislation is vital for the health of Americans. Sidestream smoke kills up to five thousand people a year through lung cancer; it produces chronic lung obstruction, and other major diseases in thousands of other people. Tobacco's effects are like a time bomb; work in an office with smokers and twenty years later, you may become a grim statistic in an epidemiologist's notebook.

Sidestream smoke causes all sorts of short-term problems, too: eye irritation appears in 70 percent of nonsmokers, and headaches, nausea, and coughing are prevalent in about 20 to 30 percent of people trapped around smokers. There's also the fact that cigarette smoke is extraordinarily annoying. Passive smoke is irritating—it can quickly ruin a pleasant dinner out, or make the workplace something to loathe.

Laws banning smoking in public places and the workplace should be pursued with the same vigor as other public health measures such as campaigns to contain tuberculosis, drunk driving, AIDS, and drug abuse because like these disorders, *passive smoking kills*. It's deadly. Passive smoking is a public health menace as great as any that faces the country—and states must be required, through legislation, to take the action necessary to save people's lives.

That's the purpose of nonsmokers' rights legislation.

In much of the country there still are no laws regulating smoking. And in much of the country there are conflicts between smokers and nonsmokers. Smokers want to smoke, but nonsmokers want to breathe air that is as safe as possible—or have to if they have allergies or asthma. At restaurants nonsmokers become irritated when, halfway through their meal, someone lights up at the table next to them. Smokers are bothered by people asking them not to smoke after they've already put a match to their cigarette. Nonsmokers have to ask their fellow workers not to smoke, or ultimately complain to their supervisors, to their managers, or to the head of their companies (who, in the absence of guidelines, may not be equipped to resolve these problems)—and this only breeds dissension. Pregnant women and people with allergies must avoid cigarette smoke or constantly have to tap smokers on the shoulder and plead, "please don't smoke." Some smokers are twisting their heads from side to side, trying to calculate whether the people around them are going to ask them not to smoke; other smokers are becoming arrogant and obstinate about their habit. Instead of courtesy, conflict is becoming increasingly common between smokers and nonsmokers; ambiguity creates confusion and unpleasant encounters. The absence of clear guidelines on where smoking is prohibited forces the issue to become a conflict between smokers and nonsmokers.

Courtesy is bound to fail when there are strongly opposing interests. That's the theory, a theory which is borne out by evidence: Smokers light up just about wherever they want, even though 86 percent of nonsmokers believe that smokers should refrain from smoking in the presence of nonsmokers. A smoker says to himself "I'm gonna smoke and if somebody objects, let him say something." The burden of courtesy is placed on the nonsmoker, for whom the issue is not one of courtesy, but of health.

Common courtesy also falls apart because smoking isn't just a "habit" (see Glossary, Appendix C) or a pastime, but a real physical and psychological addiction. Asking someone not to smoke is like asking heroin or cocaine addicts to hold off on their "habit" when their minds and bodies crave the drug. It's arduous to stop smoking temporarily; it takes more than courtesy to stop smoking.

For nonsmokers, having to ask smokers to refrain from lighting up is a continual burden.

As nonsmokers, we're often intimidated out of asking a nonsmoker to stop. It takes chutzpah and occasionally more to ask a smoker to put his cigarette out. Indeed, sometimes, nonsmokers' worst fears about asking a smoker to refrain are justified. Human behavior is unpredictable, and who wants to take the risk that a smoker will lash out or strike the nonsmoker verbally—or physically? Not the New York City off-duty police officer who was shot in the face without any warning after he asked a youth not to smoke in a no-smoking car in Pennsylvania station. The police officer was in plain clothes and did not identify himself as a cop; he asked the youth not to smoke, just as an average citizen might.[1]

In Richmond, Virginia, a man asked a woman not to smoke at a Wendy's restaurant. He waved his hand to push her smoke away. The woman, who worked for Philip Morris, decided that she would claim the man hit her cigarette out of her mouth, and had him charged with assault. (He was found not guilty.)

Nonsmokers simply shouldn't be forced into dangerous, awkward, or disturbing actions.

Besides smoothing relations between smokers and nonsmokers, laws that ban smoking are money-savers, too. They save money in two ways. First, they help employers and restaurant owners—by reducing health, fire and life insurance premiums, dramatically cutting cleaning and furniture replacement costs, and by making workers healthier. Healthy employees are productive employees. Every one less smoker saves his employer between $500 and $1000 a year over the long term; and for every nonsmoker who is no longer exposed to tobacco smoke in the workplace, another $50 to $100 a year is saved. Even waiters who serve tables with smokers stand to gain by no-smoking regulations. Second, smoking places a fantastic burden on the American economy as well as on state and local governments. The tune of this cost is about $11 billion a year in health care costs, or a total of $930 billion since the Surgeon General's first report on smoking was published in 1964. (And these figures do not count property damage, maintenance, lost earnings, decreased productivity—an estimated $53 billion a year in all.)

The struggle for nonsmokers' rights "is a battle between health and greed," said Ahron Leichtman who successfully passed ordinances to curtail public smoking in Cincinnati. "It is the health of all . . . versus the greed of the tobacco companies."

What Kind of Legislation Should You Pursue?

There's a wide range of possible laws that you can lobby for. At the weaker end of the spectrum are laws that merely empathize with the problems that nonsmokers face, and recommend courtesy or bar smoking in places such as hospital halls and school classrooms. The strongest laws prohibit smoking in all workplaces and all public places.

As we will see, there are plenty of ways to structure these codes. Your efforts should be directed toward enacting the most restrictive law possible, not only because it is the best in terms of public health, but because it may be the easiest to pass. Many states and localities have been able to pass extremely pro-nonsmokers' rights laws.

In general, laws that ban smoking affect two different arenas: the workplace and public places. The latter can include public transportation, taxis, restaurants, hospitals, movie houses, theaters, concert halls, retail stores, waiting rooms, auditoriums, government buildings—virtually everywhere that people gather. It's possible to propose two separate sets of laws, one pertaining to the workplace and the other to public places, but in practice it makes much more sense to aim toward restricting smoking in both. The focus of any nonsmokers' rights legislation should be to protect the health of nonsmokers (a category that includes former smokers, of which there are a million new ones a year). Only by including both the workplace and public places can these laws truly protect people's health. Excluding one or the other continues to make people vulnerable to tobacco smoke. Most states and localities that have enacted nonsmokers' rights laws have combined the workplace and public places in the same legislation.

A valuable resource for figuring out how to write the legislation is your local Board of Elections. The board can provide information on how referenda and legislation are passed, who legislators are, from whom they receive their campaign funds, and when they are next up for election. This information will help you set the stage for a successful legislative campaign.

What Legislation Looks Like

Laws need to be precise, and that's one of the reasons why laws seem so complicated. A detailed law will reduce the possibility of evading the law. Fortunately, laws restricting smoking are usually not as complicated as other laws. Moreover, excellent laws banning smoking have already been enacted—so writing legislation isn't much more difficult than adapting one of the successful models to your area. Appendix B contains two model ordinances.

Parts of Smoking Restriction Laws

Laws regulating smoking have numerous parts, or in legalese, sections. Refer to the sample nonsmokers' rights codes, as you read the descriptions that follow. The San Francisco legislation is an excellent example of workplace smoking restrictions, and the San Diego law provides a strong model of an overall bill; both should be emulated.

Affected Sections of Code

The first part of your bill should specify what section of code is affected by this proposed legislation. In most cases your bill will amend a particular part of your city or state's laws, and this section of the bill says into what part of the law the bill will be incorporated, as well as what laws are changed by the bill. A proposed nonsmokers' rights bill may affect more than one section of established code.

Title

The bill's title should be something that describes the legislation's intention. This section won't cause too much controversy (compared to other sections, anyway); the Smoking Pollution Control Ordinance is fine to use.

Findings and Purpose

This explains why the legislation is required and what the law is supposed to do.

Explain the detrimental effects of smoking on nonsmokers and talk about particular subgroups of nonsmokers, including people with allergies, asthma, lung disease, eye problems, pregnant women, and children. This discussion does not have to include statistics or references to particular studies, but it can. The statements about the health effects of involuntary smoking should be clear and unequivocal. You should then say that the City Council or State Legislature declares that the purposes of this act are to 1) protect the health and welfare of the citizens by prohibiting smoking in public places except where specifically exempted and 2) to balance the *desires* (definitely not "rights") of smokers to smoke with the *need* of nonsmokers to breathe unpolluted air. It's also important to point out that *in the event of a conflict or ambiguity between smokers and nonsmokers, "no smoking shall have priority,"* or *"the rights and needs of tobacco-smokefree air shall have priority,"* or as stated in the San Francisco legislation, *"if a satisfactory accommodation cannot be reached, to prohibit smoking in . . ."* (Emphasis added.) This theme, that nonsmokers' rights must prevail when there's a disagreement about whether smoking should be allowed in a particular environment, should be embodied throughout the legislation.

Definitions

This section says what you mean. Every important action, object, or place has to be precisely defined. Definitions may be a subject of controversy. Whether you narrowly or broadly define a particular place, for example, can affect how many people are protected by that law. You will need to define terms such as city, state, person, smoking, to smoke, public place, retail tobacco store, employer, employee, business, workplace, home, dining area, restaurant, bar, enclosed area, theater, motion picture theater, hospital, health care facility, sports arena, waiting area, and service line. Some of these definitions can be grouped together under the categories business or workplace.

Application to Government Facilities

Does the law apply to municipal or state-owned buildings? It should.

Prohibitions and Designations of Smoking Areas in Public Places

This is the nitty-gritty section of the legislation. Here the bill says exactly where smoking is not allowed. The San Diego bill provides the simplest prohibition, and the best: "No person shall smoke in a public place or place of employment except in designated smoking areas." The San Diego bill then lists under "Designation of Smoking Areas" those places in which there *may not* be smoking areas. The San Diego law is very specific about where smoking areas may not be located, but also leaves open the possibility of banning smoking in areas not specifically mentioned by the bill. This is important: You want to declare certain areas *no smoking*, but not limit your bill to those areas. An alternative is to write, "No person shall smoke in a public place *with the following exceptions* . . . ," and then the exceptions can be enumerated. If you follow this approach, you should also point out that the fire marshal or public health commissioner has the authority to nullify these exceptions.

You may have to get fairly specific in describing what kinds of facilities are covered. For restaurants, it's necessary to describe what size restaurants are affected (by number of seats or square feet), whether bars are included, and how smoking and no-smoking areas should be divided. For theaters, restaurants, and other meeting places, you should specify whether private functions are covered. The ordinances in Appendix B provide good guidelines for this.

Places in which there should be no smoking—ever—include hospitals, senior citizen centers, nursing centers, banks, polling places, public rest rooms, elevators, taxis, retail stores, arenas, convention centers, public meeting rooms, government buildings, jury rooms, court houses, indoor public transportation waiting areas, airports, and where there is a fire hazard. Places in which there ought to be at least 50 percent no smoking—assuming adequate ventilation—include restaurants and theater lobbies.

The bill should also state that any facility may be designated entirely a no-smoking area by employers or store owners. All the legislation does is set a minimum standard.

Prohibitions and Designations of Smoking Areas in Places of Employment

The same prohibitions should be specified for the workplace. It's a good idea to separate the workplace and public places into different sections, because this makes the bill less complicated. It also makes it easier to modify in the event that there's overwhelming opposition to the bill by one special interest, say restaurant owners. You can then change that section without watering down the rest of the legislation.

San Francisco's municipal code requires employers to provide a no-smoking work area to any employee who objects to smoking around her. The employer is required to try to accommodate the smokers and nonsmokers through ventilation, partitions, and separation, but not required to spend any money at this task. If a compromise between smokers and nonsmokers cannot be made, the needs of the nonsmokers will take priority. Even if just one nonsmoking employee objects, that employee will be granted a nonsmoking workplace.

A better regulation would be to prohibit smoking in all work areas, rather than allowing employees to designate no-smoking zones where they work. Even with a clause that bars employers from retaliating against employees who speak out for their rights, some nonsmoking employees may feel uncomfortable insisting on their rights. (Workplaces that are 100 percent smokefree report no problems between smokers and nonsmokers.)

Again, your legislation should be open enough to allow employers to implement stricter restrictions, such as having a completely smoke-free workplace and hiring only nonsmokers.

Nonretaliation

It's important to put into law that any employer who fires, demotes, harasses, or refuses to hire an employee or applicant for exercising her rights under this law is in violation of law. You should specify separate penalties for this. In addition, you may want to write into existing local law that it is illegal to retaliate against people for exercising their rights under this law.

Where Smoking Is Not Regulated

In order to prevent the nonsmokers' rights legislation from creating hardships, it should list exceptions and exemptions. For example, sole proprietorships (one-person offices), though workplaces, ought not to be included in the bill. The same goes for private homes used as workplaces. In the spirit of compromise, you may decide to make an exception for tobacco retail stores, private social functions, and hotel rooms. The bill should also allow individuals and businesses to apply for a special exemption because of unique conditions or hardships. Your bill can specify that an exemption can be granted only after a public hearing is held to determine whether it would be a financial hardship for that organization to comply with the law.

Timetable

The bill should specify a date or timetable for implementation. The schedule for the starting dates of public smoking restrictions and for workplace smoking restrictions need not be the same. Your legislation needs to spell out a date by which employers have to announce their new policies to employees. This information can be placed in a separate section or within the sections on prohibitions.

Posting Signs

Signs are just about the only enforcement tool that smokers' rights laws need. An attractive, simple *No Smoking* sign or universal no-smoking symbol, a smoldering cigarette inside a circle with a diagonal red slash through the middle, is all you need to implement the law. People are good about obeying no-smoking signs—better, in fact, than they are about obeying red lights and no-littering laws.

The Smoking Pollution Control Ordinance must specify where no-smoking signs are to be posted. Entrances, in rest rooms, staircases, lobbies, and inside meeting halls are good locations for no-smoking signs. You should describe what the signs ought to look like, and what the minimum size is. In addition, movie theaters ought to be required to display a no-smoking message on the screen for five seconds before the movie starts.

Enforcement and Appeal

Usually the director of public health or city manager is responsible for enforcing the regulation. The fire department may also inspect for violations, but complaints should not be directed toward that agency unless smoking constitutes a fire hazard. Citizens may complain to the director of public health or city manager and initiate enforcement of the law.

The director of public health or city manager should provide new license applicants with copies of the bill, as well as answering questions about the regulations.

Business owners and managers are required to post the no-smoking signs. The bill may also point out that they are required to inform people verbally who are violating the law that they should stop smoking.

Violations and Penalties

This is the least used section of any nonsmokers' rights legislation, because there are hardly any violations once the law takes effect. But you should say that it's unlawful for any person covered by the bill to fail to comply with its restrictions. Any person who fails to post a no-smoking sign, inform someone that he is in violation of the law (as per above section), or who violates the law, shall be fined 1) not less than $10 dollars and not more than $100 for the first infraction, 2) not more than $200 for the second violation of this bill within one year, and 3) not more than $500 for each additional infraction within one year. You should specify whether each day a violation occurs will be considered a separate infraction under the code.

Education

The bill should stipulate that the director of public health or the city manager embark on a program to explain the law. You may want to specify that a pamphlet shall be printed to guide citizens toward complying with the law. The bill can say whether the director of public health and city manager should also strive to educate people about the dangers of involuntary *and* mainstream smoking. Because these education campaigns are inexpensive, it isn't necessary to write into the bill a budget for this (or for enforcement).

Government Agency Cooperation

This section ensures that the policy is communicated to and implemented in other departments of the municipal or state government. It requires the city manager, governor, or director of public health to educate other agencies about the law and establish procedures for cooperating with it. It should also urge enforcement of the law in agencies of other governments, such as federal or state offices, that do business in the jurisdiction in which the law applies.

Other Applicable Laws

In this section there should be a sentence saying that this article shall not be construed to permit smoking in places where it is restricted by other laws, such as regulations under the city's fire code.

Servability

This means that if a part of this bill is found to be invalid that will not affect the validity of the rest of the bill.

Legislative Dangers

There are worse things that can happen to your bill than not passing. If the legislation is defeated, you can try again next year; and next year will be easier because the most difficult part of the process will have already been accomplished—putting the idea into people's heads. But if a weak bill is passed, you will have a tremendously difficult time convincing legislators to introduce stronger measures. They will have suffered one fight and won't be relishing another.

These weakening measures are called nonsmokers' rights legislation killers. Watch out for them. You can be certain that the tobacco interests will try and slip them in.

The most dangerous clause is "Nothing in this section (or article) shall prevent designation of the entirety of any facility as a 'smoking' or 'no-smoking' area." This phrase will probably be the first that the cigarette interests try to introduce to see how far they can go. A confidential report prepared by the Roper Organization in 1978 recommended "The industry might propose that operators of restaurants, cabs, and other public 'institutions' be permitted to establish whatever smoking policy they desire—'Smoking permitted anywhere,' 'No smoking permitted,' 'Separate facilities for smokers,' or 'Separate facilities for nonsmokers,'—but with the requirement that the smoking conditions that apply be posted outside the premises for the convenience and protection of smokers and nonsmokers alike.'' *Beware:* this sentence cancels the entire bill; it makes the legislation worthless; it gives any employer, restaurant owner, or manager the ability to say that smoking is allowed. The only acceptable variation of this sentence is: "Nothing in the section (or article) shall prevent designation of the entirety of any facility as a *no-smoking* area."

In Chicago, smoking is banned in meeting rooms and taxi cabs. The city's law requires restaurants with more than forty seats to have nonsmoking sections. Workplaces must have no-smoking areas if employees want them. Bars and private meetings are not covered by the law. New York's law is strict and is working fine. Restaurants with fifty or more seats must create no-smoking sections. In workplaces with more than fifteen workers, employees may designate their work area as a nonsmoking area. But if smoke drifts into no-smoking areas, the employer must make "reasonable" additional changes. Smoking is prohibited in classrooms, rest rooms, and common areas. Retail stores that have room for more than one hundred-fifty shoppers must bar smoking. In hotels, 50 percent of the lobby area must be declared off-limits to smoking, and there can be no smoking within twenty-five feet of the front desk. Smoking is prohibited in taxicabs.

Legislation enacted by the Pennsylvania legislature in 1988 is an example of a weak law. Only restaurants seating more than seventy-five people have to have no-smoking sections, and the proprietors can determine the relative sizes of these sections. In contrast, other states, such as Minnesota, require no-smoking sections to be separated by a physical barrier at least fifty-six inches high *and* have certain types of ventilation *and* maintain certain minimum carbon dioxide standards. Pennsylvania's new law says that employers must develop policies to regulate smoking in their workplaces, but the law does not specify what these policies must look like. In Michigan's workplaces smokers must find smoking sections; in Pennsylvania, it's up to the nonsmoker to locate a safe place to breathe. The premise of the law is to "protect the public health and to provide for the comfort of all parties by regulating and controlling smoking in certain public places and at public meetings and in certain workplaces." Compare this with the preamble to New Jersey's nonsmokers' rights law: "The right of the nonsmoker to breathe clean air supersedes the right of the smoker to smoke." But the most disturbing part of Pennsylvania's bill is its preemption clause that causes the law to supersede any town's stricter antismoking laws. Preemption clauses are dangerous. The preemption clause prevents any other city from enacting a stricter law.[2]

Preemption also ruined West Palm Beach's no-smoking law. Between 1980 and 1985 West Palm Beach had a strict nonsmokers' rights law that was disemboweled when the state legislature passed a "Clean Indoor Air Act," a much weaker law than Palm Beach had.

The Tobacco Institute has plenty of tricks up its sleeve. During the debate over the proposed legislation they're bound to argue that implementing the law will be expensive. They'll point to the costs of purchasing no-smoking signs, modifying offices and other structures to comply with the new law, the cost of informing people about the law, hiring inspectors, and the additional burden on the courts. The Roper report again: "*While the public widely supports government programs to discourage cigarette smoking,* a majority opposes spending tax dollars for such a program—which suggests such programs might be vulnerable if people were made aware of their costs." (Emphasis added.) As we'll see in a moment, in every place where there are nonsmokers' rights laws the total costs have been minimal, and in the long run the laws have actually saved money. However, the cigarette companies will try to promote this falsehood and suggest that the bill incorporate a clause that prohibits the expenditure of *any* money associated with this legislation. They may propose something like, "No city (or state) funds may be appropriated or spent directly or indirectly in conjunction with any part of this article." And that may seem to make sense, because proponents of the legislation insist that the consequences of the legislation won't cost much. However, there are always some costs, usually indirect, associated with any legislation, such as printing the regulations, involving overtime of an already-hired government employee, answering queries, printing an informational brochure, sending letters, and yes, purchasing no-smoking signs.

Prohibiting *any* money from being spent on the law makes it impotent. And in the long run it costs *more* money as the costs of smoking in the workplace and public places continue to escalate.

If that tactic doesn't work, the Tobacco Institute may try to bar funds from being spent on educating people about the law. They may suggest wording to the effect: "No funds may be appropriated directly or indirectly on educational or informational purposes with regard to this article." Education—the truth—is the real enemy of the cigarette companies. The more people know and understand about the human and economic consequences of involuntary smoking, the more they will oppose smoking in public. But the tobacco interests may ask, "Why should environmental tobacco smoke be singled out for extra expenditures for unnecessary education? It's just another waste of money, especially in times of tight budgets." (Of course they'd never use the same terminology about subsidies to tobacco farmers or regarding the deductibility of tobacco advertising expenditures.) Stress the points that educating people about nonsmokers' rights won't be expensive, and that it is important to let people know about the law. Governments usually try hard to inform people about a law that requires some change in behavior. Mandatory seat-belt, drunk-driving, and pooper-scooper regulations (that require dog owners to pick up after their pets) are three examples of public health and safety laws that state and local governments have spent considerable time educating their citizens about.

The "Definitions" section of the bill is a tempting place for the tobacco interests to try to weaken your law. It's likely that they will attempt to define the "place of work" as an indoor area in which fifty or more persons are employed. Clearly, this is an unacceptable proposal, because it excludes smaller businesses and will force tens of thousands of people to be needlessly exposed to tobacco smoke. The law should be applied fairly to all people; it is supposed to protect everyone. Better to say, as the San Francisco statute does, "If an accommodation which is satisfactory to all affected nonsmoking employees cannot be reached in any given office workplace, the preferences of nonsmoking employees shall prevail and the employer shall prohibit smoking in that office workplace." Or, "In all places of work smoking shall be prohibited in all work areas."

The same tactic may be tried with restaurants. It is to the advantage of the Tobacco Institute to exclude restaurants that seat fewer than a hundred persons, and to exclude restaurants that have their bar and dining area in the same room. For all practical purposes this can mean all restaurants will be excluded. If your legislation is encumbered with this kind of wording, it's better not to deal with restaurants at all for the present, and to try again later, after everyone has had a chance to witness how successful the law has become in other places.

If your bill proposes to make it illegal to smoke on any form of mass transportation, including private buses, vans, and taxis, you should look out for clauses that say it's okay to smoke at the back of these vehicles. Ventilation is never good enough to keep tobacco smoke from waffling forward, and the people sitting in the seats nearest the smoking section will invariably be exposed to high concentrations of tobacco smoke. In addition, some nonsmoking riders will occasionally be forced to ride in the smoking section of a crowded bus, van, or train. (We know. Bill Adler, Jr., traveled from Denver, Colorado, to Flagstaff, Arizona, by bus once, a twenty-hour ride. It was a ten-pack-a-day ride.) An acceptable compromise is to allow smoking on trains only in a separate smoking car, and only if there are five or more cars on the train, and the smoking car is not also the snack or dining car.

At the behest of the tobacco interests a city council member or state legislator may attempt to exempt rest rooms, lobbies, waiting areas, bus and train depots, or hallways. These are used by everyone, and these places frequently have poor ventilation and no windows. Any effort to make exceptions for these areas should be opposed.

Bad legislation is also legislation that does not require *no-smoking* signs. Signs are the most important tool for informing people where they cannot smoke—and without them the bill is not worth passing.

The same is true for penalties. Even though fines will hardly ever be levied, there must be sanctions for disobeying the law—otherwise it has no teeth. It is the *threat* of a penalty, coupled with the desire of people to obey the law, that makes it work. Fight any effort to strike or weaken the provision in your bill for penalties.

A voluntary law, of course, is the worst possible legislation. Self-regulation is what already exists and doesn't work. The issue is public health and it should not be treated trivially—thousands of lives are at risk. However, voluntary legislation can be acceptable if there is absolutely no chance of a real law passing *and* it is written into the bill that if the voluntary regulations do not work, then mandatory legislation will automatically be considered. The voluntary law should also state the criteria for determining whether the law is working and should specify the language of the actual bill.

State Versus Local Legislation

You will have to decide whether to pursue legislation on the state or local level. Obviously, a statewide campaign is more difficult, more expensive, and more likely to raise the ire of the tobacco companies. The Tobacco Institute will spend hundreds of thousands *or millions* of dollars fighting nonsmokers' rights laws in a state. It's easier for them to concentrate on fifty states than it is to spread their resources around thousands of city and county campaigns.

A statewide campaign will be a media campaign. GASP should only attempt to pass a nonsmokers' rights bill in the state if you have a combination of ample money, strong supporters in the state house or governor's office, significant editorial support, a large grass-roots organization, the active support of public health, medical, insurance, fire fighters, or related groups, and political skills. A statewide legislative effort is easier if there are GASP groups throughout the state with experience passing laws on the local level. To fight a battle in the statehouse you will have to become more than just a volunteer organization, you'll need a paid staff and a sophisticated office. You'll be working with consultants, direct-mail specialists, lobbyists, and a range of experts. There's a tremendous amount to do to try to pass a nonsmokers' rights bill in a state, but the good news is that it's been accomplished successfully in over two dozen states.

Referendum Versus Legislation

As you progress toward introducing legislation to support nonsmokers' rights you may be stymied by yet another tobacco tactic: calling for a referendum. Some state legislators may also support the notion of letting the people vote on whether to have laws against smoking in public. If there's one thing that politicians hate, its being forced to vote on controversial issues, because no matter what they do, they are going to alienate some voters. The tobacco industry favors a referendum because referenda are easier to influence—they can bring the full power of their propaganda machine into play. A referendum lets the tobacco industry spend countless dollars on media, not to mention brochures, sophisticated surveys, and getting out the vote. The side with the most money is at an advantage during a referendum: They can con voters into believing that nonsmokers' rights legislation would be discriminatory, expensive, promote lawlessness, be the stepping stone for banning other "personal habits," and isn't necessary. But in legislatures, each of the cigarette companies' arguments can be met by an equally loud—and more honest—counter argument.

In a legislative battle you will be able to focus your attention on a smaller number of legislators. Some will already be on your side, some opposed; it's the so-called swing votes you will have to convince. On the other hand, with a referendum you won't have any idea which voters are in your camp without expensive polling.

This is not to say that referenda always fail. They have succeeded in places like San Francisco (though not the first time around). And most people do want restrictions on smoking in public places. But the tobacco industry has more experience, more consultants, and more money to fight a battle for the hearts and minds of voters.

Referenda are supposed to be rare birds, too. They should be used sparingly, reserved only for the most fundamental constitutional issues. Nonsmokers' rights is a public health and safety concern. Legislatures are competent at dealing with this kind of issue, and should.

Are No-Smoking Laws Constitutional?

Whenever you introduce nonsmokers' rights legislation you'll hear some voices loudly proclaim that antismoking laws are unconstitutional. Sometimes these utterances come from smokers who are afraid that the legislature is going to take away their "right" to smoke, sometimes from legislators and lawyers who should know better, and almost always from the Tobacco Institute (with the help of their lawyers). One legal opinion, prepared by the firm Brodovsky, Brodovsky & Grossfeld for the tobacco side, concluded that the Sacramento nonsmoking legislation would be "not only unconstitutional on its face but would be unconstitutional in its application. Moreover, the enforcement provisions are clearly violative of the protections afforded a criminal defendant both under the Constitution and under the laws of the State of California. Finally, a practical application of the law would not only be unworkable and a burden on private industry but also would result in the hopeless congestion of our local courts."[3]

Of course, the results of Sacramento's law turned out just the opposite of Brodovsky, Brodovsky & Grossfeld's opinion. It's in place and perfectly constitutional.

Fortunately, nonsmokers' rights legislation is constitutional, standing on firm, legal ground; it has not been successfully challenged in court.

Cities and states are allowed to regulate smoking in public places as long as these laws do not preempt higher laws, that is as long as a city's restrictions do not contradict state law and as long as state laws don't run counter to federal regulations. (If there is a conflict, the higher law is the authority in the absence of a court opinion.) But although these regulations may not "preempt" higher laws, they may be more restrictive than existing laws. As long as a particular body such as a city council, board of supervisors, or state legislature has the authority to pass general laws—legislative power—it has the legal authority to make laws on smoking in public places. Councils' and legislatures' powers extend into many areas; usually the statute that establishes these bodies specifically says they can make laws to preserve public safety and health, and to prevent injury to the public. Outdoor air pollution has been a frequent target of city and state laws in the past; now it's indoor air pollution's turn. In addition, states and municipalities frequently have the authority to pass laws affecting occupational health and safety. Public safety and health have always been defined broadly because new public health problems can't always be anticipated when the legislation is created. That's why legislation dealing with nonsmokers' rights is introduced by a section explaining the dangers of passive smoking. Indeed, if the Tobacco Institute wanted to question the constitutionality of nonsmokers' rights laws they would have to challenge in court the premise that involuntary smoking is harmful. Notice how they have not done this.

A United States Supreme Court decision about a regulation on a local smoke-pollution code (*Huron Portland Cement Co.* v. *Detroit*, 1960) said:

The ordinance was enacted for the manifest purpose of promoting the health and welfare of the city's inhabitants. Legislation designed to free from pollution the very air that people breathe clearly falls within the traditional concept of what is compendiously known as the police power.

Opponents of nonsmokers' rights say that these laws violate the equal protection clauses of the U.S. Constitution, the Fourteenth Amendment. Tobacco attorney Grossfeld's words again:

It is a well-established principle that the Equal Protection Clause prohibits state and local governing bodies from enacting laws which contain classifications that are arbitrary and without rational relation to the interest sought to be advanced by the law . . . .

For example, certain businesses are faced with a total prohibition against smoking, such as stores, banks, terminals, and buses and taxis. Others, such as offices, theaters, arenas, recreation halls and restaurants, have a partial smoking prohibition. Still others . . . are exempt from the ordinance.

Grossfeld is wrong. The Supreme Court and the Constitution allow classifications to be made as long as they are not "purely arbitrary." It recognizes that distinctions among people, places, or actions will be made under law. The Court ruled, "The equal protection clause of the 14th Amendment does not take from the state the power to classify in the adoption of police laws, but admits of the exercise of a wide scope of discretion in that regard . . . ."[4] These classifications do not have to be made with "mathematical nicety." This judicial reasoning applies not only to places where smoking is banned or restricted, but to people as well. Nonsmokers' rights laws do not arbitrarily deprive people of their personal liberties, but balance, as the law provides, the desires of people to pursue certain activities and the dangers those activities have on others.

State and federal courts, including the Supreme Court have continually upheld the notion that businesses do not have the privilege to engage in unrestrained or unregulated activities. Time and time again courts say that it is the province of legislatures to make laws governing the activity of businesses, because courts do not have the expertise to develop procedures for regulating them. In other words, the judiciary upholds the authority of the legislature to pass laws regulating any number or kind of businesses.

Do Smoking Laws Discriminate?

There are two fears concerning nonsmokers' rights laws. First, that they are by their nature discriminatory, and second, that they may enable an employer to use these laws as a way of discriminating against blacks, hispanics, and other minorities.

As we've seen, although nonsmokers' rights laws do separate smokers and nonsmokers, they are not legally discriminatory. However, are these laws ethical? The answer is yes, because they don't segregate people on the basis of any intrinsic quality such as race, religion, national origin, sex, or anything visible at all. Smokers aren't shier, taller, rounder than nonsmokers (however, many have stained teeth and bad breath, but these maladies are a product of smoking, not of who the smoker is). *The distinction these laws make is not between people, but between actions.* Anybody can enter a no-smoking area and stay there as long as he wants. The only criterion is that he not smoke a cigarette. Smokers can even enter no-smoking areas holding cigarettes in their hands or mouth, as long as the cigarettes aren't lit. Neither the philosophy nor the substance of the law is aimed at smokers. *It's not smokers who are offensive, but tobacco smoke.* There's no animosity between smokers and nonsmokers, especially because a lot of nonsmokers are either married to smokers, friends with smokers, or the relatives of smokers.

There's a second element to the Tobacco Institute's smoking-laws-discriminate argument. They contend that because more blacks smoke than whites—43 percent to 35 percent for adult men, 33 to 30 percent for women—that antismoking laws *ipso facto* are discriminatory. Blacks are disproportionately affected by laws that prevent smoking and this is unfair, they say. The Tobacco Institute carries the argument one step further: More blacks are in lower-paying outer-office jobs than whites, and when antismoking laws allow smoking in private offices, frequently occupied by whites, but not in public spaces such as reception areas where more blacks work, that's doubly unfair.

These arguments are fallacious. Really good nonsmokers' rights laws prohibit smoking everywhere in an office—in both the private and public spaces—because cigarette smoke travels freely throughout a building. The second-best laws allow any worker, black or white, to demand that her workplace be smokefree. It may be that more blacks than whites smoke, but there's an important converse that the Tobacco Institute conveniently ignores—57 percent of black men and 67 percent of black women do not smoke. Black nonsmokers deserve to be protected from toxins in tobacco smoke just as much as whites do. And even though blacks smoke in larger proportions than whites, there are, on average, more whites in the workplace than blacks, so more white workers are affected by smoking regulations than blacks. Either way, insisting that nonsmokers' rights laws discriminate is absurd. Smoking has nothing to do with being black, hispanic, Italian, white, Jewish, Catholic, or anything at all (except from the cigarette companies vantage point; they see blacks as a growing market).

Tobacco companies also like to dredge up the argument that telling blacks they shouldn't smoke is paternalistic at best, racist at worst, because more blacks *do* smoke than whites. Scott Stapf, former assistant to the president of the Tobacco Institute, said, "To me that is a racist approach." But the nonsmokers' rights movement isn't concerned about whether people smoke or not—nonsmokers only want smokers to refrain from lighting up around them. Black doctors, just like white doctors, say that smoking is dangerous. What's especially obnoxious is that the Tobacco Institute is *using* racism to defend smoking. Something former Secretary of Health and Human Services Joseph Califano said about women who smoke can also be applied to blacks: "Women," he warned, "who smoke like men die like men." Lung cancer is color blind.

The notion that antismoking laws could be used by employers who want to discriminate is also absurd. Not a single case of an employer using nonsmokers' rights laws to discriminate has been filed. The tobacco industry likes to pack smokers into the same category as minorities which have truly been victims of discrimination. Ed Larson, of the State Retail Tobacco Dealers' Association, said, "We hear constantly about the discrimination. We cannot discriminate against whites, blacks, gays, people with AIDS, but we can discriminate against cigarette smokers."[5] Discrimination is a problem—it is evil—

but trying to link nonsmoking law with discrimination only detracts from efforts to stop it.

Opponents of Nonsmokers' Rights and Countering Their Arguments

You're not going to make friends with your entire community by fighting for nonsmokers' rights. There are plenty of groups—other than the cigarette companies and their hired hands—that oppose legislation on smoking. Once the legislation is on the books, many of the people who opposed the bill will be fully behind it, but that prospect doesn't help you at the onset.

Nonsmokers' rights legislation cuts across party lines. There are Democrats and Republicans who support the idea, and there are members of both parties who think that antismoking laws are stupid; the same goes for liberals and conservatives. Smokers, of course, oppose the regulations more than nonsmokers, although not always vehemently or cohesively. (Many smokers are looking for help in quitting and many prefer not to get in a situation in which they might annoy a nonsmoker).

Groups that are likely to oppose any effort to pass nonsmokers' rights legislation include restaurant owners, restaurant associations, legislators who smoke, hotels, some unions, taxicab drivers, business owners, and cigarette merchants and distributors. Plus any prominent individuals or public relations companies and other firms paid by the Tobacco Institute.

The most certain opponents are the Tobacco Institute and other organizations involved in selling cigarettes. These include vending-machine operators, trucking companies, small stores that receive much of their income from the sale of tobacco products, billboard owners, advertising companies, and possibly local publications that receive a large percentage of their advertising budget from cigarette companies. (Chapter 1 discusses how the power of cigarette advertising influences editorial decisions at newspapers and magazines.) These are powerful and frequently desperate opponents. Their lifeblood is peddling cigarettes, and they will do and say *anything* to keep as many people smoking as often as possible.

The tobacco industry is going to spend plenty of money and buy as many allies as possible. How much money? In 1988 the industry spent $3 million to defeat legislation in Oregon that would have banned smoking in all indoor public places except tobacco shops, some hotel rooms, and bars.

There isn't much you can do to change the minds of tobacco organizations. However, you can weaken their positions and arguments. Because you are on the side of the angels, you can speak freely to voters or legislators about how the tobacco groups are only concerned about money. Talk about the money the cigarette companies make. Explain that the trend toward eliminating indoor air pollution through nonsmokers' rights legislation is one of the most dangerous threats the tobacco companies are facing because it not only directly reduces their income, but makes smoking socially unacceptable, like spitting. Laws that ban smoking in public places say, "Smoking around others is wrong—and there's something wrong about smoking, too." These laws, the tobacco companies are deathly afraid, won't just reduce the number of cigarettes that people smoke each day, but will decrease the number of smokers overall and stop new smokers from being initiated. Estimate how much money cigarette companies earn in your city or state each year and mention this figure as often as possible. Point out that the tobacco companies don't care about health, which is also true. Place side-by-side 1) the statements of the Surgeon General, the National Institutes of Health, and the American Cancer Society that say that smoking causes cancer, heart disease, lung disorders, and fetal damage, along with 2) the evasive denials by the Tobacco Institute that there's no "proof" smoking is harmful. Ask your legislators, "If the cigarette companies won't even admit that *mainstream* smoking is harmful, how can you believe *anything* they say?"

Knock down the tobacco industry's lies. The tobacco companies will lie subtly, or blatantly, but lie they will. For example, in California the tobacco interests published a brochure which said:

> Claims that nonsmokers' health is endangered by other people's smoke are contradicted by many physicians who speak for the antismoking organizations. Dr. Jonathan Rhoads, past president of the American Cancer Society, said, "I do not have any hard evidence [that there is a harmful effect from

sota Department of Health has been receiving an average of about 137 complaints per year from nonsmoking employees involving alleged workplace violations. Virtually all of these complaints have been resolved satisfactorily through correspondence and discussions between Department personnel, the employer, and the employee. To my knowledge there have been no lawsuits involving workplace violations."[8]

And what about the costs? What about the charge that smoking restrictions break the budgets of states and municipalities? Here's how the health officer of the City of Pasadena answers that question: "I have no figures on enforcement costs since no account was set up to handle them. There are costs, I'm sure, but they are minimal at best."[9] In San Francisco: "Initial manpower requirements entailed the use of one inspector on a full-time basis in order to handle the large amount of requests for information and complaints. The amount of time spent on matters related to the Smoking Ordinance has gradually declined to a current level of approximately one day per week."[10] San Jose, California, estimates that "the smoking regulations have cost the city less than $80.00 per month."[11]

Criminals do not roam the streets because the police are too busy enforcing antismoking laws. In most localities the public health department, not the police, enforces smokers' rights laws. The police are not hampered by these laws. Nonsmokers' rights laws have zero effect on crime.

Typically, the forces opposed to nonsmokers' rights legislation use names like "Committee for Common Courtesy" in New York City, "San Franciscans Against Government Intrusion," or "Californians for Common Sense." These names are as shadowy as the arguments the tobacco companies use. These organizations are not comprised of a "committee" of people who believe in common sense, or "Californians"; rather they are funded directly and heavily by the tobacco companies. The Tobacco Institute has regional groups, but these, too, are funded from Washington, and ultimately, they all receive their money from the tobacco companies. The Tobacco Institute never reveals its political budget, so it's going to be difficult to calculate how much money they're spending. In fact, their employees are not allowed to disclose their salaries. But we know that the Tobacco Institute spent $1.25 million in San Francisco against nonsmokers' rights legislation in 1983; four years earlier they spent $1.1 million in Miami. Each cigarette company contributes to the campaign in accordance with its market share. The Tobacco Institute and cigarette companies will deny being directly involved in the campaign, even though they control the misnamed citizens' committees. They may acknowledge making minor contributions, but will never admit to financing the pro-smoking groups. It's worthwhile trying to uncover how much the tobacco lobby is spending. If your state requires lobbying organizations to file reports relating to political activities, some of their expenditures will be public, though not all. When you learn which law, advertising, and public relations firm the Tobacco Institute has employed, call these companies to find out their rates. Next, make some rough estimates about printing costs, television and radio advertising time, office space, transportation, and so forth. Look hard for other consultants and expenditures. Add these figures and you will have a rough idea— undoubtedly an underestimation—of how much the Tobacco Institute is spending to defeat nonsmokers' rights legislation. Remember, unlike the proponents of nonsmokers' rights, the Tobacco Institute doesn't rely on volunteers—everyone on their side is paid and paid well.

The Tobacco Institute insists that the majority of people don't want laws on smoking, and it conducts periodic polls to prove that assertion. But these polls use weighted questions that bias people who are surveyed toward particular answers. For example, a Tobacco Institute-sponsored poll conducted in 1984 in Los Angeles asked whether nonsmoking laws should be enforced "aggressively" by police, or by lawsuits against employers, without offering any benign choices. This poll also asked questions that included phrases such as " . . . because employers and employees should determine a company's policies, not the government." The survey discovered that 41 percent of the public thought the L.A. City Council should just urge businesses to adopt no-smoking sections, and 39 percent thought the City shouldn't become involved in any way. But unbiased polls, such as those conducted by the Gallup organization in California in the same year as the tobacco-sponsored poll, showed that 77 percent of all adults want no-smoking sections in restaurants (16 percent want it banned altogether) and 70 percent of the public wants smokers segregated in the workplace (16 percent think it should be banned). That's the difference between an honest and biased poll. But what's amusing about the Tobacco Institute polls is that a private survey conducted for them by the Roper organization in 1978 concluded that "There is a majority sentiment for separate smoking sections in all public places we asked about." Here's what that majority looked like:

PLACES FOR RESTRICTING SMOKING

Trains, airplanes, and buses	91 percent
Theaters	83 percent
Eating places	73 percent
Indoor sporting events	73 percent
Public meetings	67 percent
Train, plane, and bus stations	62 percent
Workplaces and offices	61 percent
Barber and beauty shops	53 percent

Source: Roper Survey for the Tobacco Institute, 1978

The figures that the Tobacco Institute obtained in its secret poll mirrors those obtained by Gallup polls. For example, 23 percent of respondents said smoking should be *banned* in restaurants and 17 percent thought it should be *banned* at public meetings. And on the issue of how phrasing questions during a survey affects the answers, the Roper report said, "Had we asked about banning before mentioning the acceptable alternative of segregation, the sentiment for banning might have been substantially higher." Remember, too, this poll was conducted in 1978 and the public attitude toward smoking has swung much more in favor of nonsmokers' rights since then!

The Tobacco Institute isn't bashful about publicizing falsehoods. In full-page advertisements placed in *The Washington Post, The New York Times*, and other papers in January 1989, the Institute said, "Enough Legislation! A majority of Americans do not support smoking bans according to a national poll." In a footnote the Tobacco Institute cited a poll conducted by Hamilton, Frederic & Schneiders. Several newspapers obtained the actual results of this poll and found that *according to the Tobacco Institute survey* 74 percent of respondents favored separate smoking and no-smoking sections, while one fourth of the people who were surveyed supported banning smoking altogether in restaurants.

Once these laws are enacted, the percentage of supporters is even higher. Berkeley, California, enacted its tough antismoking laws in

1977. A year later, when a statewide referendum was considered to ban smoking in public places, 61 percent of Berkeleyites supported that referendum, despite the tobacco industry's multimillion-dollar campaign to defeat it. Minnesota also provides a testament showing how people like nonsmokers' rights legislation. Eight years after the Minnesota Clean Indoor Air Act passed, *92 percent* of all adults in the state—including smokers and nonsmokers—supported restricting smoking in public places including the workplace, restaurants, and other public places.

Local surveys frequently show that extremely large numbers of citizens want nonsmokers' rights strengthened. These surveys often give numbers that are higher than the national averages. Citizens of Waynesboro, Virginia, who live in tobacco country, favor restrictions on smoking in enclosed public places by an 88.2 percent margin! A whopping 90 percent want separate smoking and no-smoking sections in restaurants![12]

Tobacco's closest allies, such as billboard owners, cigarette distributors (who are usually also candy distributors), vending-machine companies, and some retail outlets that sell cigarettes, will also be in the forefront of trying to defeat smoking restrictions. They may participate by contributing to the "Committee for Common Sense" or whatever it's called, or they may be more actively involved. Some of these groups may also be from out of state; when this is the case you should make that point loud and clear. These businesses will have been told by the tobacco industry that they stand to lose a lot of money if nonsmokers' rights legislation is passed. This isn't true, because nonsmokers' rights doesn't prohibit smoking, it simply prevents people from smoking where they can harm others. You don't see the alcohol companies screaming because drinking isn't allowed in public, neither have the makers of large portable radios (not-so-affectionately known as boom boxes) raised a furor over some cities' laws (including New York's), which prohibit them from being played on the street.

The billboard companies are always good allies of the tobacco industry. After all, they receive most of their income from cigarette advertising. R.J. Reynolds is the number one billboard advertiser in America, Philip Morris is number two, Brown & Williamson (makers of Kool) is number four, and American Tobacco is number six. However, the billboard companies really have nothing to do with the question of nonsmokers' rights, because this legislation doesn't affect billboards. But what the activity of these businesses in the nonsmokers' rights campaign does is demonstrate the ability of the Tobacco Institute to call in favors owed.

Many restaurant and hotel owners (other than the growing number who offer no-smoking sections) and their respective associations are bound to vehemently oppose restrictions on smoking in their establishments. They're concerned, as anyone would be, that new regulations could harm their businesses. Pat Olson of the New York State Restaurant Association expresses the typical concern: "The demand for 50 percent of restaurants to be off-limits to smokers just isn't there. This is going to mean lines, waiting, and loss of business. We're going to see restaurants close."[13] Basically that's hogwash. Nonsmokers' rights legislation helps businesses cut costs.

The fears of restaurant owners are quickly alleviated. Here's what *The Washington Post* reported about one locality:

When Fairfax County decided to restrict smoking in restaurants, business persons braced for the worst: Empty tables in no-smoking sections; costly renovations to comply with the new law; county health inspectors watching intently for errant diners to light up.

But after living with the regulations for seven weeks, many once-skeptical restaurant operators are surprising even themselves with their reaction. They say it has been easy to implement and that their customers are enthusiastic about the law.

"We're constantly amazed at how successful it has been," said Noel Panella, assistant general manager of Clyde's of Tysons Corner. "The nonsmoking rooms are continually full, and the clients are very happy. It's really proved a point to the restaurants in that it has presented no problems.

"At first we were very leery about it," Panella said. "We were afraid it would cut down on our flexibility and hurt business . . ."

Gregory T. Farell, manager of Chi-Chi's restaurant in Springfield, Va., applauds the regulation. "I think it has helped business. People really appreciate that we offer it," he said. "We have proven the doomsayers wrong . . ."

One of those who initially had reservations about the Fairfax ordinance is Douglas T. Wilson, manager of Charley's, a 185-seat restaurant . . . Wilson said he and others were concerned about the potential costs of installing ventilation systems and erecting barriers, as well as with the prospect of long lines of patrons waiting for seats to open in the smoking sections.

"It's really not as bad as some people thought," Wilson says now . . .

At Chi-Chi's in Springfield, Farell said, the public response has been so positive that owners of the Mexican-American restaurant have reserved 65 percent of the 480 seats for nonsmokers . . . [The law requires 25 percent.]

"All the feedback I'm getting from people [in the restaurant business] seems very favorable," said Panella of Clyde's. "The managers are amazed at how full their restaurants are."[14]

One restaurant in Portland, Oregon, offers a 15 percent discount to patrons who sit at nonsmoking tables. That's certainly indicative of how no smoking cuts costs for restaurants.

Associations that represent restaurants and businesses are ideologically opposed to any restriction imposed by law. Chambers of commerce fit into this category, too. The essential premise of business associations is that the Government Shall Not Regulate. Even in the face of absolute success, as in Fairfax County, restaurant associations will not acknowledge the sense of nonsmokers' rights. They're fearful and jumpy, like city squirrels. In the words of James Wordsworth, president of the Northern Virginia chapter of the Virginia Restaurant Association: "If you allow this to happen, then what's next? We're more concerned that it's going to open the gates [to more regulations]." Michael Kidwell, manager of Joe Theismann's restaurant in Virginia, maintains, "There is no doubt in my mind that cigarette smoking is not healthy, not only for the people who are doing the smoking but also [for] the people surrounding it. I think the big issue here, however, is overregulation." It is in that philosophy—the danger of sliding down a slippery slope of government intrusion—that opposition to nonsmokers' rights is often born. It's a close-minded view, and your job is to prevent that philosophy from becoming contagious.

Nonsmokers' rights laws do not lead to overregulation. It is axiomatic that regulations are conceived independent of other laws, debated and passed by legislatures. One kind of regulation does not make it more likely that another will be passed. In fact, most legislatures are set up so that laws are very difficult to pass. In most states, and the U.S. Congress, only a tiny fraction of bills introduced ever become law.

As of late 1988, twenty-three states have enacted laws requiring restaurants (of a certain size) to set aside no-smoking sections. At least two cities, Palo Alto, California, and Aspen, Colorado, completely ban smoking in restaurants.

Restaurant owners (often through their louder compatriot, the Tobacco Institute) say that if patrons wanted no-smoking sections, they would demand it. This is the *marketplace fallacy*, the argument that the marketplace can determine whether no-smoking sections are desired. There are some important problems with this argument. The marketplace should not decide public health problems. We don't let the marketplace decide about outdoor air pollution, and shouldn't let it determine the quality of air indoors. The issue is health—not preferences. When it comes to health, governments are obligated to protect people. Witness laws requiring children who are riding in cars to be fastened into child safety seats; laws regulating the removal of asbestos from buildings; and mandatory immunizations for children entering school. Governments have a special obligation to protect people; volunteerism isn't sufficient where lives are concerned. When the New York City Department of Health asked restaurants to voluntarily set aside 25 percent of their seats for nonsmokers, only 3.5 percent said they would. As an editorial in *The New York Times* said, "Asking restaurants voluntarily to create a nonsmoking section, then, is about as effective as asking people not to park on the street. It's the *threat* of a fine, not the call to honor that works . . . Courtesy having failed, it's time to try clout."[15] (Emphasis added.)

But if the marketplace were the determining factor as restaurant associations say, how should it be measured? The technique preferred by businesses is a market survey, asking potential customers about their preferences. Well, the latest market survey, a 1987 Gallup poll, says that 77 percent of all adults and 86 percent of all nonsmokers (the plurality of the population) want smokers to "refrain from smoking in the presence of nonsmokers." *A 1984 Gallup survey of 1,038 adults found that being exposed to cigarette smoke was among the top five reasons why people don't eat out more often!* Thirty percent of all adults said that it was "very true" they didn't eat at restaurants more often because of smoking, and 17 percent responded that it was "somewhat true." Another technique used to determine people's preferences is to establish a focus group, letting a collection of consumers try a product and see how they react. This experiment can be performed by just about anyone: Ask a bunch of nonsmokers who've been eating at tables next to smokers whether they enjoyed that smoke. Then ask nonsmokers who have been dining in a smokefree environment if they prefer that to a smoky restaurant. The answers will be clearly overwhelming on the side of no smoking in restaurants. Many restaurateurs who have either voluntarily or involuntarily set aside no-smoking sections, have found that a no-smoking section that occupies 50 percent of their space just isn't large enough to accommodate all the people who want to sit in the no-smoking area. Plenty of smokers don't like tobacco fumes spoiling their meal, either, and so they, too, rush to the nonsmoking sections—as a result, many *nonsmokers* never get a seat in the no-smoking sections.

When Bill Adler, Jr., debated Walker Merryman of the Tobacco Institute on WRC Radio in Washington, D.C., he asked sardonically, what's magical about setting aside 50 percent of a restaurant's seats for nonsmokers? Why 50 percent? Well, 50 percent no smoking—the most common arrangement among cities with smoking restrictions— isn't magical. It's reasonable. For too long nonsmokers have had to put up with zero no-smoking seats; that's unfair and unhealthy. Better than 50 percent, however, would be to reserve 75 percent of a restaurant's seats for nonsmokers, in accordance with the Gallup survey's results. Or 100 percent no smoking. That's even healthier and surely smokers can go without a cigarette for an hour or so.

The health problem is the big issue surrounding smoking at restaurants, as it is in any public place. But tobacco smoke is also annoying and it is more disturbing at restaurants than anywhere else. It ruins the taste of meals. No, more accurately it makes food smell and taste like tobacco. Which is the same thing as ruining a meal.

Restaurant owners are afraid that banning smoking (the ideal but rarest solution) will annoy their best patrons. It may, just as deciding not to allow cigar or pipe smoking—the norm in many restaurants— temporarily upset some smokers. But cigar and pipe smokers have managed to survive an entire meal without smoking, and so will cigarette users. A 1983 Gallup poll said that only the teeniest minority of smokers (13 percent) believe (*before* legislation is passed) that there should be no restrictions on smoking in restaurants. And most of these minds change after regulations are in place. Restaurateurs are worried that some patrons will no longer be able to sit at "their" table if it's in the wrong section. This is a silly and condescending attitude toward people. Nonsmokers and smokers breathe easier when there are clearly marked no-smoking sections. Nonsmokers, and the vast majority of smokers who eat out, enjoy unpolluted air and the ability to smell their duck à l'orange, chablis, and white chocolate mousse; smokers will tell you that it's a pleasure to go through a meal without being glared at by a nonsmoker or worrying about whether one's going to be asked, "would you mind not smoking, please?"

Owners of restaurants are afraid that laws regulating smoking will send patrons elsewhere. But when *all* restaurants are regulated equally, all restaurants are on an equally competitive footing. The law takes away any fear of unfair advantage.

Restaurant owners are concerned that no-smoking sections will force them to install walls, partitions, or expensive air scrubbers. They take a hysterical view of the law. But nonsmokers' rights bills require no such things. Most legislation specifically says that business owners do not have to incur any expenses in meeting the law, except for buying a few No Smoking signs.

The savings are considerable. Restaurants may be places of entertainment for patrons, but they are workplaces for waiters, and the less tobacco smoke waiters are exposed to, the less they are absent from work. Restaurant smoking restrictions cut down on the number of ashtrays restaurants have to replace and clean. Carpets are easier to maintain. These laws mean fewer curtains to replace, and few unattractive little burns in tablecloths. Fire and health insurance rates decline. The bill for maintaining the air conditioners is smaller.

But best of all: Diners like separate sections. In an article reporting on the effects of New York City's antismoking law, *The New York Times* reported, "Six months ago, a significant number of New York's restaurateurs were ready to tear their hair out as the city's new smoking law went into effect." (The law requires restaurants that have more than fifty seats to divide their space into separate smoking and nonsmoking sections.) The *Times* continued, "Now the same restaurateurs who were predicting disaster admit, a bit sheepishly, that none of their dire predictions have come true." Pay attention to the words of one restaurant owner quoted in the *Times*: " 'We were overemphasizing the difficulties in the beginning because we wanted regulations we could live with,' said Tony May, owner of the Palio . . . Now Mr. May, who has set aside the front of his restaurant for nonsmokers, said, 'No problem. The regulations were written in such a manner that we were able to live with them quite well.' "[16]

Smoking and eating out are not inextricably linked—that's just a tobacco industry myth. When smoking and eating out do not mix, everybody's happier.

Many businesses, those that dwell in office buildings in particular, will oppose laws that prohibit smoking or banish it to distant cubicles. They argue about the costs, the difficulty of enforcing and monitoring these laws, the paperwork (they have enough already), the burden to taxpayers, how it discriminates against blue collar workers, who comprise the majority of smokers, how it isn't necessary, how it singles out their business. Bear in mind, that while these are legitimate concerns, they are unfounded. Business owners already enforce many workplace safety laws with ease. Laws to regulate smoking are actually egalitarian because they apply fairly to all places of work. When there is no ambiguity over where smoking is allowed, conflict between nonsmokers and smokers is replaced by harmony: Both sides understand the rules. Nonsmokers feel better because their health is protected, and smokers are relieved that they won't be hassled about their habit anymore. Reducing smoking at work cuts back on absenteeism and dramatically reduces the costs of doing business.

Nonsmokers' rights laws are among the only regulations that actually save both businesses and the taxpayer money.

And these laws work brilliantly. Michael Smith, an epidemiologist at the University of California reports that San Francisco's law on smoking in the workplace, the toughest in the country, "has been one of the biggest non-events in San Francisco."

John Angius, a spokesperson for Pacific Gas and Electric, which employs seven thousand people, said of San Francisco's law, "It has gone incredibly well. The few problems we've had were solved by moving some furniture around."[17]

NOTES

(1) *The New York Times,* January 2, 1986, p. B3.

(2) "Anti-smoking Bill Leaves Many Huffing, Many Puffing," *Philadelphia Inquirer,* November 27, 1988, p. 1.

(3) Sheldon H. Grossfeld to Jack Kelley, legal opinion letter, Tobacco Institute, November 20, 1984.

(4) *Lindsay v. Natural Carbonic Gas Co.,* 1910.

(5) *Town Meeting,* KOMO-TV, Seattle, October 26, 1986.

(6) Californians for Common Sense brochure, 1978.

(7) "County close to being smoke-free," *Contra Costa Times,* November 17, 1984.

(8) C. B. Schneider, chief, Environmental Field Services, Minnesota Department of Health, letter to Dr. Raymond Weisberg, president, San Franciscans for Local Control, September 26, 1983.

(9) Dr. Elton Blum, letter, August 1, 1985.

(10) Bruce Tsutsui, inspector, central office, Department of Public Health, City of San Francisco, letter, May 16, 1985.

(11) Rita Hardin, director, Neighborhood Preservation, letter to Sylvia Jutila, chair, American Cancer Society, August 16, 1985.

(12) Waynesboro League of Women Voters, 1987 survey.

(13) "Nassau Restaurants Facing Strict Limits on Diners' Smoking," *The New York Times,* November 7, 1985, p. A1.

(14) *The Washington Post,* April 3, 1987.

(15) *The New York Times.*

(16) "The Smoking Law Revisited: Room Enough for Everyone," Marian Burros, *The New York Times,* October 12, 1988, p. C4.

(17) "County close to being smoke-free," *Contra Costa Times,* November 17, 1984.

CHAPTER 5

Enacting Nonsmokers' Rights Laws Part II: Allies and Tactics

In contrast to the liquor industry, which trumpets the virtues of moderation, the tobacco industry has never publicly acknowledged its products have any risks. But most smokers know the risks only too well and feel a smoldering resentment about their addiction. So in trying to mobilize them, the industry has had to divert their attention from its product and the merits of smoking.

Alix M. Freedman,
The Wall Street Journal,
April 11, 1988

Allies

Fighting to enact nonsmokers' rights laws is a time-consuming, emotionally, physically, and financially draining task. But if that description seems daunting remember this: Nonsmokers' rights are something you can win. And when you win, you will have clean, healthier air to breathe. Although opponents of nonsmokers' rights represent rich and powerful special interests, you will always have plenty of supporters, including average citizens. Your most important organizational allies are the health groups such as the American Lung Association, the American Heart Association, and the American Cancer Society. These organizations have been involved in fighting against tobacco smoke for decades, and have a vastly different objective than the cigarette companies—saving lives. They have experience, expertise, and determination. If you're working on a statewide campaign, these health organizations will already be involved; but they're not always aware of local initiatives. Get in touch with the national, state, and local chapters of these groups.

Most other health and medical organizations are on the side of preventing disease from cigarette smoke, too. That includes individual physicians and the American Medical Association. These organizations and people may not fathom how they can help pass nonsmokers' rights legislation, so you will have to tell them what you're doing, why it's important, and what they should do. And they can help in plenty of ways. First, mere endorsements by people in the medical community are useful. It won't take long for the lineup of pro- and anti-nonsmokers' rights sides to become apparent: Pro- are the doctors and health groups; anti- are the cigarette companies and firms that rely on tobacco dollars. Physicians have tremendous credibility on medical issues, so the more doctors who lend their name to your cause, the better.

Second, ask these groups and individuals for contributions. Doctors groups and physicians themselves—especially cancer and pulmonary specialists and pediatricians—are an excellent financial resource.

Third, it's worthwhile forming a subgroup of your GASP called Pediatricians for a Smokefree Society, or Cancer Specialists for Safe, Tobaccofree Air. Medical doctors can assist your lobbying campaign directly by writing letters, visiting city council members, and speaking before other organizations. But you will have to approach each of these groups and cajole them into participating. As any good lobbyist knows, half the time spent lobbying is used to coax other people and groups into becoming lobbyists for your cause.

Insurance companies' support of nonsmokers' rights is particularly upsetting to the Tobacco Institute because ordinary people look at insurance companies and wonder, what do *they* have to gain by supporting nonsmokers' rights. The answer is simple: The fewer people who smoke and the fewer nonsmokers exposed to tobacco, the less benefits insurance firms have to pay. It's impossible for the Tobacco Institute to impugn the motives of the insurance companies by saying, "Insurance firms just care about their profits, that's why they don't want people to smoke," without drawing attention to their own profit-seeking motives. Insurance companies may not want to become involved in this effort, because their clients are both smokers and nonsmokers, but some forward-looking firms will. Many insurance firms restrict or ban smoking in their offices, so regardless of whether they want to campaign actively with you, you can include on your literature the names of those insurance companies that already have the same kind of restrictions that the law is seeking to impose.

Businesses and restaurants that already have no-smoking regulations are potential allies, too. These firms have *proven* that nonsmoking restrictions work well and work easily. Businesses and restaurants may contribute financially, publicly lend their names, testify before the state legislature, lobby individual legislators—their experiences are very persuasive—and write op-ed articles in your local papers. But even if they won't actively become involved, you can use their positive experiences with nonsmokers' rights in your campaign literature. Interview these companies; ask restaurants how quickly the nonsmoking sections fill; ask businesses whether their insurance or absenteeism rates have dropped and whether nonsmokers and smokers are happy. It's wonderful when local businesses demonstrate that smoking regulations are economically, medically, and socially beneficial.

More Allies

Celebrities are important allies. Athletes, entertainers, and news anchors are often staunch nonsmokers' rights activists. They're worried about their appearance (not fond of nicotine-stained teeth or clothing that smells like a used ashtray) and their health. Athletes are opposed to anything that interferes with their performance. Some celebrities get real mad when forced to breathe cigarette smoke. Sam Donaldson, ABC News' White House correspondent, is a nonsmokers' rights crusader. He's campaigned for a nonsmoking section in the White House press room. (Donaldson quit his twenty-three-year, pack-and-a-half-a-day habit in 1971.) Celebrities are often vocal and articulate, respected and listened to. They can get into state legislators' offices more easily than the average citizen (a sad, but true commentary on the nature of politicians), and have little trouble finding their way in front of television cameras. And sports figures, movie stars, and authors usually are more astute and honest than tobacco spokespeople. Some celebrities who detest breathing tobacco smoke may be willing to appear on radio and television commercials in support of nonsmokers' rights.

Politicians and civic leaders can also be instrumental in lobbying for nonsmokers' rights. Like athletes and entertainers, many find tobacco smoke disgusting. But politicians have an added incentive to support your legislative campaign: According to the 1978 Roper poll conducted for the Tobacco Institute, "More people say they would vote for than against a political candidate who takes a position favoring a ban on smoking in public places." The Tobacco Institute and related businesses contribute heavily to political campaigns and buy a lot of influence through advertising and by sponsoring sports and other events. But once politicians realize that they stand to gain more votes (in addition to doing the *right* thing) by supporting nonsmokers' rights, you may have an easier time coaxing them along. Even if a particular politician isn't going to vote on the bill, it's useful to have her support; for example, getting the mayor on your side while the city council is debating nonsmokers' rights can convince city council members that they ought to vote for nonsmokers' rights legislation.

Another major ally will be the public health commissioner. Usually a physician and often trained in epidemiology, health commissioners are stalwart supporters of nonsmoking restrictions. Many have the ability to operate independently of the city or state government, just as the Surgeon General can issue statements and take actions without the approval of the President, who appoints him. Get in touch with the health commissioner early in your campaign; the commissioner's office may have experience dealing with the city council and may be able to provide you not only with advice, but invaluable clout. Attending press conferences, meeting with council members, issuing statements to rebut Tobacco Institute arguments are only some of the roles health commissioners can play.

Environmental organizations concerned with outdoor air pollution have a stake in keeping indoor air clean, too. Numerous environmental groups have worked on issues involving asbestos, formaldehyde, and indoor spraying of pesticides. While these groups are already overwhelmed with work and probably won't be able to lend you any staff, they can help by endorsing your campaign and by providing expertise. Their years of experience battling powerful industries, and winning, can be extremely valuable. Environmental groups know the political paths well and have numerous contacts in the media and political communities: Ask them to introduce you to their friends.

Fire departments are potentially strong allies. Smoking is a grave fire hazard. In 1981 there were 59,000 residential fires, 3,445 people who were burned so severely they had to be hospitalized, and 1,622 deaths—all caused by smoldering cigarettes. In 1983, 1,270 people died from cigarettes that ignited mattresses, bedding, and upholstered furniture. Fire departments are in the forefront when it comes to adopting policies of hiring only nonsmokers. Alexandria, Arlington, and Fairfax County, Virginia; Janesville, Wisconsin; Manteca, California; Midwest City, Norman, and Oklahoma City, Oklahoma; Salem, Oregon; and Wichita, Kansas, are some of the fire departments that don't hire smokers.

Unions are potential allies, as well, but you may have to work hard to get them on your side. Labor hasn't always been a champion of nonsmokers' rights, and this is disappointing; sometimes they've even supported tobacco's positions. But there are progressive labor organizations and you'll have to approach each individually.

And, occasionally, smokers are strong supporters of nonsmokers' rights. Not all smokers are misologists who blindly follow the Tobacco Institute's pseudophilosophy. Those smokers who stand with nonsmokers' rights do so for three reasons. First, they believe that while smoking is a choice, nonsmokers should not have to inhale potentially harmful cigarette fumes. Second, they view nonsmokers' rights laws as a way of helping them break their addiction. For example, Charles Graves, who works for the Cincinnati city government, said about the city's no-smoking ordinance, "I think it helped me quit. I don't have any real big problems with it."[1] Third, smokers don't like being asked not to smoke when they light up; nonsmokers' rights laws eliminate that problem.

Using the Media

The press is like a sophisticated gear; it enables you to multiply your capacity for doing work. Through the press you can inform people about nonsmokers' rights, obtain new members, debate issues, coax reluctant legislators to your side, and expose the lies of the Tobacco Institute. But the media is more than a tool, it is vital. Although 77 percent of all adults (including 64 percent of all smokers) support nonsmokers' rights, it doesn't always appear this way to local legislators. Cigarette companies are practiced at getting their message across, and have the ability to transform their limitless dollars into voices.

Once you introduce nonsmokers' rights legislation, reporters will automatically become interested in what you are doing, but you won't automatically be presented in the best light. You will have to curry the press's favor.

Press releases are the mainstay of what you'll be feeding the press, although, just like bread, press releases alone won't keep your effort alive. The caveats concerning press releases are just as important as their benefits. Too many organizations rely on press releases to attract reporters to their events. Press releases are used as a *secondary* means of informing reporters about your activities. Secondary because reporters are deluged daily by press releases. Reporters also don't like to rely on releases for their articles, because most are one-sided. *USA Today* business reporter Mark Lewyn said, "It takes me a couple of hours just to sort through all of them in the morning. Most of them are garbage, though some are useful because they have good tips." What you do put in your releases must look sharp and read perfectly. Reporter Lewyn again, "Too many press releases are written more poorly than high school term papers."

Put some quotable remarks in your release. Give reporters something they can use directly in their articles. Releases should tell who is doing or saying what, when, and where. They should always include the most important information in the opening sentences.

Be sure to mail your press releases in time. Don't rely on the postal service to get them there the next day.

Press releases can be used for alerting the press to such events as introducing legislation, holding rallies, announcing nonsmoking dances, for countering Tobacco Institute propaganda (such as explaining the nonscience behind their polls), letting the press know about the latest developments in research on the health effects of involuntary smoking, and announcing endorsement for nonsmokers' rights legislation. Below are two mock press releases created for this book:

Vermonters for Nonsmokers' Rights

55 Maine Avenue
Montpelier, VT 02394

FOR RELEASE
December 1, 1989

Contact: April Tanner
(o) 555-3432
(h) 555-2983

NONSMOKERS' RIGHTS LEGISLATION INTRODUCED TODAY

City Council member Janice Celeste today introduced a bill to protect nonsmokers from tobacco smoke in the air. The Comprehensive Indoor Air Pollution Act restricts or bans smoking in most indoor spaces where the public meets—including city buildings, movie theaters, offices, hospitals, train and bus stations, restaurants, and schools.

"This legislation will help protect the residents of Montpelier from the harmful constituents of tobacco smoke," said Jane Kreskill, president of Vermonters for Nonsmokers' Rights. "While it's been known since 1964 that smoking causes disease, only more recently have studies proven that passive or involuntary cigarette smoking is harmful," Kreskill added. A 1984 study estimated that between 500 and 5,000 nonsmoking Americans die each year of lung cancer because they are exposed to cigarette smoke. Hundreds of thousands of others experience disorders such as headaches, coughing, burning eyes, and allergic reactions, and heart and lung diseases. Children who are exposed to cigarette smoke have a significantly higher rate of pneumonia and bronchitis.

Sidestream smoke contains 4,000 chemicals, including nicotine (a heart stimulant), carbon monoxide (which interferes with the blood's ability to carry oxygen), polonium-210 (a radioactive element), and dimethylnitrosamine (a potent carcinogen).

The Surgeon General, National Academy of Sciences, Office of Technology Assessment, and numerous other prestigious medical and scientific groups have labeled passive smoking a threat to health. "People have the right to breathe clean air indoors and out," Kreskill said.

"We estimate that positive smoking kills between 75 and 150 people in Vermont each year," she added.

Smoking is also expensive. "Death, fires, and absenteeism from involuntary smoking costs the state's economy over $50 million each year." Studies have found that smokers cost their employers about $350 a year in increased absenteeism, insurance, damage to furniture and equipment, and lost productivity. In addition, each nonsmoker exposed to tobacco in the workplace adds $50 a year to his employer's costs.

"Our proposed legislation is modeled after successful legislation in San Francisco, Suffolk County, New York, and the state of Minnesota," said Kreskill. She also pointed out that although many people are initially concerned that legislation to restrict smoking may be expensive, hard to enforce and promote disharmony, just the opposite is true. "We've studied effects of nonsmokers' rights laws and found that not only are they universally accepted and inexpensive to enforce, but they actually save money by reducing costs associated with smoking."

The Comprehensive Indoor Air Pollution Act would prohibit smoking in all city buildings, theaters, rest rooms, elevators, staircases, hospitals (except for designated lounges), bus and train waiting rooms, retail stores, and schools. The bill would also allow a single nonsmoking employee to designate her workplace a nonsmoking area, and would require restaurants that seat more than 40 people to set aside 50 percent of their seats for nonsmokers. Fines are $10 for the first offense, $25 for the second, and $50 for the third offense committed in a six-month period.

Also supporting the bill are Councilmembers Bill Morrison, Sandy McKenna, and Austin Rogers. The Montpelier Fire Department, and the local chapters of the American Lung Association, American Heart Association, and American Cancer Society are backing the legislation, as well.

Vermonters for Nonsmokers' Rights was founded in 1984. It is a nonprofit organization dedicated to protecting nonsmokers from involuntary tobacco smoke. Already Vermonters for Nonsmokers' Rights has succeeded in passing nonsmokers' rights legislation in Bromley, Stratton, and Woodstock.

(See attached sheet for more information on passive smoking and health.)

Vermonters for Nonsmokers' Rights

55 Maine Avenue
Montpelier, VT 02394

FOR IMMEDIATE RELEASE
March 4, 1990

Contact: April Tanner
(o) 555-3432
(h) 555-2983

VERMONTERS FOR NONSMOKERS' RIGHTS PRESIDENT CALLS TOBACCO INSTITUTE STATEMENT "A LIE"

VNSR president, Jane Kreskill, blasted the Tobacco Institute for calling involuntary cigarette smoking "a nonissue." Ms. Kreskill said that the Tobacco Institute assertions that "passive cigarette smoking isn't a health problem" and "we can deal with whatever controversy arises through simple, common courtesy" are utterly false.

Ms. Kreskill pointed out that the conferences cited by the Tobacco Institute which purport to show that there's no evidence that passive smoking is harmful, were actually sponsored by the cigarette industry. "The Tobacco Institute quoted papers presented at these two conferences. Papers are not the product of careful studies and peer review; anybody can present a paper at a conference. And that's exactly what tobacco's supporters did."

She added, "The Tobacco Institute's term 'claimed risks' is a variation of newspeak—*smokespeak.*

"We know for certain that passive cigarette smoke is harmful, and, according to the National Academy of Sciences, especially dangerous to children. Their 1986 report concluded, 'Since children exposed to ETS [environmental tobacco smoke] from parental smoking have an increased frequency of pulmonary symptoms and respiratory infections, *it is prudent to eliminate ETS exposure from the environments of small children.*' [Their emphasis.]

"The Tobacco Institute hasn't even acknowledged that mainstream smoking is harmful," Kreskill added. "So how can you believe anything they say at all?"

The Office of the Surgeon General, National Academy of Sciences, the Ontario Medical Association, and the Canadian Medical Association Journal, have concluded that passive smoking can be harmful. These are reputable scientific groups with nothing to gain from taking positions on passive smoking and health, she said. The Tobacco Institute's motives, however, are guided by the need to sell cigarettes, she pointed out.

"Vermonters for Nonsmokers' Rights believes that on issues of public health and safety—especially where the majority of the population is at risk—the government should take an active role to protect people. 'Common courtesy' is a nice sounding phrase, but it means that nonsmokers, whenever they want to breathe unpolluted air, must take the initiative by asking someone to put out their cigarette. So-called common courtesy only breeds ambiguity, dissension, and disease," Kreskill said.

The Comprehensive Indoor Air Pollution Act doesn't ban smoking, but restricts it in public places. Vermonters for Nonsmokers' Rights believes that this is a reasonable compromise between the desires of smokers to smoke, and the rights of individuals to safe air.

Developing contacts in the media is good practice. Reporters are people, too, and it's beneficial for you to become friendly with them. Early in your campaign you ought to identify the reporters at the television, radio stations, and newspapers who will cover the non-smokers' rights beat—they could be on the city desk, business section, health reporters, or in general news—and get to know them. Find out the names of the hosts of the local talk shows, too. Put together reference kits on passive smoking, health, and business for these reporters. Send your materials directly to those individuals; call them up from time to time when you have timely information. But don't pester them with frivolous information; don't try to persuade reporters, lobby them, or give them gifts. And, above all, respect their deadline time—that's their panic hour. Keep the press informed about the Tobacco Institute's activities, supporters, and money. Invite them by phone to your press conferences. Do some reporting—the information gathering part—for them. Give the reporters the feeling that they can rely on you for accurate and up-to-date information, that you'll let them know about an event or vote well *before* it occurs. Always give them accurate information! Oh yes, send reporters birthday and New Year's cards.

Virtually all newspapers have letters-to-the-editor and op-ed pages, places for the opinions of ordinary citizens. The letters-to-the-editor page is the best place for you to complain about or compliment events affecting nonsmokers' rights. For example, if a cigarette industry poll reveals that most people do not want legislation restricting smoking, you should send a letter that day to the paper (and a press release) pointing out the deficiencies of the survey and providing contrary information. If the antilegislation group is purchasing many advertisements in the local media, your letter should explain that this group is receiving money from the Tobacco Institute in Washington, D.C., and that your GASP can't come close to matching their expenditures. Ask other GASP members as well as physicians, civil leaders, and health organizations to write letters, too. The op-ed page is a good place to present the nonsmokers' rights side of the issue in detail. To place an article on the op-ed page, call or write the editor in charge and ask if they're interested in an article about the need for legislation to protect nonsmokers. If the editor responds, for example, that a city council member has already written such a piece, explain that your article presents the citizens' perspective and will make arguments that the council member didn't or couldn't offer. Timing is important and you should aim your op-ed piece toward the week of the vote on the nonsmokers' rights bill. The op-ed page is also a good place to talk about nonsmokers' rights if the paper writes an editorial against smoking restrictions.

Television is, for better or worse, the king of media. The majority of Americans receive their news through the tube, so an effective campaign involves effective use of television.

Prepare beforehand if you anticipate being interviewed by television reporters. Preparing means having a short, exciting, one-to-five-sentence statement ready. Of course it's impossible to explain the complexities surrounding nonsmokers' rights in just a few sentences, but that's the way television operates. If you want to get on the air, your impromptu remarks should never be improvised, but carefully worded in the way that fits into television's format: concise and interesting. Think of your answers to reporters' questions as free advertising, and talk accordingly.

If a local radio or television station editorializes against your position, they will probably allow a spokesperson for your organization to present your side of the issue. Contact the station immediately in writing and by telephone and request time to reply. Your reply doesn't have to rebut the station's arguments point by point—most viewers won't remember the arguments anyway—but should simply offer GASP's views on why nonsmokers' rights legislation is needed. You may also be entitled to have your group's views aired under Federal Communications Commission requirements that radio and television stations serve the public interest, and under a statute called The Fairness Doctrine. If you believe that the station is not presenting the issue fairly, or that through advertising the tobacco side has an unfair advantage, ask the station for time to present your views. You may want to get in touch with an attorney to learn the proper procedure for following this approach. During the years when cigarette advertising on television was legal, Action on Smoking and Health's president, John Banzhaf, used this tactic to obtain free national television time—worth some $200 million—for antismoking commercials.

Every nonsmokers' rights campaign will have at least one debate, perhaps sponsored by the League of Women Voters, perhaps by a local radio or television station. Debates are inevitable.

You will have to prepare harder for your debate about nonsmokers' rights than for anything else. The Tobacco Institute will send their smoothest talkers. They will make assertions that are entirely false, but tobacco spokesmen know that words uttered on television sound true regardless of their veracity. Tobacco spokesmen will try to divert attention away from health issues toward more manageable (but irrelevant) topics like "courtesy" or "civil liberties." They will deceive the audience if they believe they can escape undiscovered.

Lobbying

Lobbying means winning legislators to your side. Successful lobbying means victory.

Step one is learning as much as you can about your legislature's or city council's process. Start by going to the library and reading articles about the history of recently passed bills and bills that failed. Talk with lobbyists who have worked on other legislation. Find out about key committees, who controls scheduling committee votes and votes of the full legislature, who the power brokers are, and everything else you can. Are the people with the greatest influence the ones who contribute to legislators' campaigns? (If yes, then you may have to enlist their support.) Does one legislator decide which bills come up for a vote? Do all bills have to go through a rules or appropriations committee? How does seniority affect legislation? Can the governor or mayor influence the process? What districts do the legislators represent? How are they apportioned? Are there at-large council members (who don't represent a specific district, but who are voted on by everyone)? How responsive are legislators to their constituents' concerns and demands? Is the legislature or council insulated from the people? Do certain legislators take their cues from others? What are the favorite subjects of individual legislators? The legislative process isn't always the way civics texts describe it; each state and city has its own, special process.

Step two is finding the best state legislator or city council member to introduce the bill. Ideally a representative on the relevant committee, such as public safety or health, is appropriate. Eventually the bill will be considered by that committee, so it is the most effective place to start. Concentrate your efforts there. The committee chairman is ideal for introducing the bill, but if the chairman isn't yet in your camp, the second best bet is one of the committee's more prestigious members.

It's important that whoever sponsors the bill be a stalwart supporter of nonsmokers' rights. The Tobacco Institute will try as hard as it can to get that legislator to abandon the legislation or water it down. Whoever the bill's sponsor is must fight for it and accept no compromises. Legislators with years of experience are more capable of defending the legislation, but some veteran legislators are, unfortunately, also accomplished compromisers. Be suspicious of the compromisers. Examine the records of the people you are considering as sponsors. Are they strong consumer or human rights advocates? Are they capable of standing up against tough lobbying by industry? Do they like to compromise, or do they insist that their legislation remains intact? Are they liked by other legislators? Are they good lobbyists themselves? What are media's attitudes toward them? What is their staff's reputation? Finally, do they have a record of passing legislation?

Not every council member or state legislator will have all these strengths, so you might consider using several principal sponsors. It helps to have both Democratic and Republican supporters—after all, the legislation is nonpartisan. Bipartisanship removes the risk of your legislation carrying excess ideological baggage. The more names attached to your legislation at the onset, the better your prospects will be.

To search for cosponsors, contact the legislators' offices and ask which staff members would be responsible for issues affecting smoking in public places, or, if they don't know, public health and safety. Write the legislator and send a copy of your letter to that staff member. Your letter should be relatively brief—no more than three pages—and should mention 1)why nonsmokers' rights laws are needed, 2)that most people support restrictions on smoking, 3)how the community would benefit from smoking restrictions, 4)the positive effects of legislation in other areas, 5)the prominent personalities in your city or state who support nonsmokers' rights, 6)about GASP and the help you will provide the legislator in writing the bill, monitoring its progress, providing information for speeches, debates and articles, and finding other cosponsors. Legislators like to know that they're not going it alone, that there are people in town who will actively support (what they see as) their legislation. Your letter should also describe why you believe that legislator is the best person to sponsor the legislation; flatter her with your knowledge and admiration for how she passed another bill—mention that bill by name. Include a one- or two-page fact sheet with quotations from the Surgeon General, National Academy of Sciences, and other organizations if you want. (You might consider including the relatively ancient, by nonsmokers' rights standards, words of the Interstate Commerce Commission, which ruled in 1971 that smoking could only take place in the last five seats of buses: "Secondhand smoke" is "an extreme irritant to humans, particularly with respect to its effect upon the eyes and breathing.") Finally, ask to meet with the legislator and her staff; then call her office the following week to set up a meeting.

Frequently the legislator who's the best potential sponsor—because she's chair of the appropriate committee and the one who oversees what the committee considers—will play hard to get. It's time, then, to marshal contacts. Find someone who knows someone who knows someone who can arrange a meeting between you and the legislator. An attorney, former council member, perhaps even a friendly reporter. Alternatively, you might request a meeting between you, the legislator, and a celebrity who's bound to impress that legislator. Or a meeting with several of the legislator's constituents (whom the legislator is supposed to represent). Whatever tactics you employ, never accept just a meeting with the staff aide. Staff, who sometimes fill the role of praetorian guards, may be hard-working, but you can never gauge how the legislator feels about an issue from the staff member's remarks. If necessary, arrange a preliminary meeting with staff, but quickly follow that with a bona fide meeting with the legislator.

The meeting will be mostly like a job interview; both parties are sizing each other up, but you want the legislator on your side more than the legislator wants you. You should impress her with your knowledge of the legislative process by talking about what phases you anticipate the bill going through, and explaining how GASP will help promote the bill. Ask questions, too: What problems does she anticipate the bill will encounter? Discuss whether the legislator will help you obtain other sponsors, or whether she feels you would be best for that. Offer an already written bill that can be dropped in the "hopper." In most cases, legislators will be pleased that they don't have to write a bill from scratch; (so will their staffs). Give the legislator a pamphlet explaining the purpose of each of the sections. Remember, you don't want the legislation changed too much—or the bill won't be worth pursuing at all.

The bill will probably be passed along to the legislature's legal council or the city attorney to insure that it conforms with the style of other laws and doesn't conflict with existing regulations. If your city council is comprised of part-time citizen-legislators, your proposed legislation may also be sent to a committee of legislators, attorneys, citizens, and local businesses to "draft" the legislation. This is a potentially dangerous step, because there's a chance that the nonsmokers' rights legislation may be watered down or stifled by these groups. There's also a possibility that representatives of the tobacco industry may be invited to participate in evaluating the legislation. If you can't avoid this process, insist that physicians and health organizations be represented, but *not* the tobacco industry. This is a public *health* issue, not a public relations project. While these ex-legislative committees are golden if they like your legislation the way it is, they are often unpredictable. So try to prevent your legislation from visiting them. As uncertain and arduous as the normal legislative process is, it's best to stick with that route. Explain to the bill's sponsor that the legislation you're proposing has already been tested in other cities and states; there's nothing experimental about the wording you've provided. It works and works well. The committee's assistance isn't needed in *drafting* the legislation. In addition, committees outside of the legislature waste time. Mention that the legislature's committee process— hearings, expert witnesses, and voting—is sufficient to examine the merits of this bill. But remember, as the legislative process progresses, *no* bill is better than a weak bill.

Talk tactics, strategies, and timetables. Discuss when hearings will be held on the bill and when the legislator expects a committee vote. This is crucial: *You don't want your bill to be introduced and never be heard from again.* Similarly, it's essential that the bill not be given perfunctory treatment by the committee. This is a common way for legislators to deal with controversial legislation, but *seem* concerned for the sake of television. They introduce legislation, go through some maneuvers, and let the bill die in committee. Only a handful of legislation ever makes it to the general legislature for a vote. You should try to get a sense of the committee's agenda and some guarantees that there will be hearings and a vote. And, throughout the process, you should stay alert to keep the bill alive. Publicity and controversy will accomplish some of this for you, but anti-nonsmokers' rights forces would love nothing more than for the legislation to suffer a silent demise.

Once the nonsmokers' rights bill is introduced it belongs to the legislator. There's a certain amount of proprietorship that's associated with legislation, and this is important to the bill's progress. The legislator's name is attached to it and so is her ego—and egos are tremendously powerful legislative forces. Let the sponsor talk about "my bill"; GASP shouldn't be crowing about the bill as *its* legislation. There will be plenty of time for praise *after* nonsmokers' rights laws are in force. The more ego the legislator has at stake, the harder she's going to push it. Let the legislator steal the show, as long as she's running the show well and not changing the program by weakening the proposed regulations.

Lobbying is more of an art than a precise science. It employs skills from public relations, acting, advertising, athletics, writing, and political science, as well as persistence and research. You can't really be taught how to lobby like you can be taught about a political system; lobbying is learned by doing. Still, there are some guidelines and techniques that you should be aware of before you start work on your nonsmokers' rights legislation.

First, and the single most important fact of lobbying, is to be completely truthful. Your credibility is your most important asset, especially as compared to the Tobacco Institute's credibility, and once credibility's gone, it's gone forever. If a report concludes that there's a range of deaths associated with passive smoking, (like the Replace-Lowrey study's five hundred to five thousand lung-cancer deaths per year), say so; don't just cite the larger figure.

Lobbying involves coaxing other people to help your cause. Capitol Hill lobbyists in Washington spend at least half their time trying to get individuals and organizations to assist their efforts. Once the bill is in the hopper, talk with your certain and potential allies; let them know that in order for nonsmokers' rights to be enacted they are going to have to become involved. It won't require a tremendous amount of their time, but it will take some. You'll have to ask them to perform specific tasks and then check once in a while to make sure they've done what they've said they were going to do.

You're probably going to be outspent by the pro-tobacco side, but that doesn't mean you're going to lose. You have to take advantage of your natural assets, which includes being a constituent. You vote, the Tobacco Institute doesn't.

GASP should write each legislator asking for their support in two ways: as cosponsors, and to vote for the bill. The letter should be short, but a one-to-two-page fact sheet can be attached. Let your most prestigious supporter sign the letter, or list the names of important, local supporters. The nonsmokers' rights bill's sponsor also needs to write each legislator and ask for their support.

One of the best ways to keep your allies—especially your members—informed is through your regular newsletter. Virginia GASP's newsletter is chock-full of information about passive smoking and health, what different groups are doing around the country, and legislative details. One issue included an "Action Alert" calling on members to write their representatives in the Virginia General Assembly. The newsletter informed its readers about the substance of the bill, which would have established nonsmoking areas in hospitals and required the posting of No Smoking signs. It also gave the bill number, said to call or write the chair of the appropriate committees, and what to say. In addition, Virginia GASP printed the names, addresses, and telephone numbers of all the members of the General Assembly. This information makes it easy for your members, and allied organizations, to take action.

After the vote, your newsletter should list who voted in favor of and who voted against nonsmokers' rights legislation. Ask your group's members to thank those legislators who supported your efforts and to chastise the representatives who said no to nonsmokers' rights. When legislators receive these letters, they'll notice, much to their chagrin, that voters actually pay attention to what they do. They'll realize their votes aren't anonymous, and perhaps vote more thoughtfully next time.

Develop a "swing chart." Each legislator or council member should be given a grade of 1 to 5, depending on his or her position toward your nonsmokers' rights legislation:

1——Definitely in favor
2——Leaning toward
3——Undecided or unknown
4——Leaning against
5——Definitely against

These fluid ratings will tell you how to apply your resources. Obviously those graded number 1 aren't in need of coaxing, other than thanking them for their support or asking them if they can help convince other members to join your side. Neither are members rated number 5 important for you to focus on. But, those rated 2, 3 or 4 are the key swing votes, the ones who will make the difference on vote-day. Remember that conversations with staff members are not necessarily accurate indicators of how a legislator thinks unless the staffer says, "I talked with the boss this morning and he said he . . ." It's vital to keep notes on what the legislators have to say about the bill throughout the campaign.

Visit as many offices as possible. When you do, bring along your famous or powerful supporters. Call legislators' offices for appointments and mention that you'll be bringing Dr. so-and-so or television personality such-and-such. Usually council members and state representatives will want to pawn you off on their staff, but if you're a constituent, or persistent and you have a notable with you, you'll get access to them.

When you meet with the legislator, start by smiling because it's contagious and potent. If you live in the legislator's district mention that. You'll probably have only five minutes to meet with him, so you should get directly to the point. Talk about the pros and cons; bring up the Tobacco Institute's arguments and then demolish them. Hone in the points that (1) this is a *local* public health issue; (2) that it will save lives; (3) that it especially protects children; (4) that it will save money for businesses and for the city; (5) that it is easy and inexpensive to enforce; (6) *that it is supported by the majority of people*—it is very popular; (7) that it resolves conflicts between smokers and nonsmokers; (8) that it is in the mainstream of thinking about health; (9) that it doesn't deprive smokers of their ability to smoke. Give the legislator a flier explaining how nonsmokers' rights legislation will work in your city or state. And don't leave without learning whether the legislator is in your camp. If a legislator says he needs time to think about it, fine; put that person in the 3 or 4 category depending on what he says, and *continue lobbying*.

In lobbying, timing is crucial; good lobbyists follow their visits not only with a personal letter, but with as many letters as possible from the legislator's constituents. After each visit, you should arrange for a dozen or more of that legislator's constituents to write to her, asking her to support the bill. This accomplishes two objectives: It lets the legislator know that her consituents care enough about nonsmokers' rights to write (and will remember how she voted come election day); and it tells the representative that your group has some influence. The legislator won't fail to recognize the political message contained in this coincidental timing. Your clout will be enhanced and the legislator will be more convinced that her constituents are behind nonsmokers' rights.

Letter-writing should be a continual lobbying tool. Concentrate on the number 2, 3, and 4 legislators and be sure that letters arrive from their constituents. Legislators don't really care about mail sent by people who neither vote for them nor contribute to their campaigns. You will have to work to get constituents to write their legislators, but the effort will pay off. Prepare an information sheet on what to write: Letters should be polite, brief, include the most important facts about passive smoking, and *urge* the representative to vote for the Nonsmokers' Rights Bill. If you write a sample letter, be sure to tell people that they should not copy that letter word for word; originality counts. Don't send postcards. Your GASP can stage a letter-writing evening where people gather to write letters over pizza.

Grass-roots lobbying should go on in other forms, too. Constituents can call their representatives and ask to talk with the legislator about the pending nonsmokers' rights bill. Petitions can be circulated and organized by groups: restaurant patrons, hospital workers, secretaries, students, lawyers, families of lung cancer patients.

As Ahron Leichtman, president of Citizens Against Tobacco Smoke, said, "Our ultimate political weapon is broad, sustained public outrage."

Intellectual persuasion isn't the only, or main, way to win legislators over to your side. Politics plays an important—sometimes key—role in this. Legislators have to perceive voting for your bill as in their interest. Will it bring them votes? Will it hurt or help their campaign finances? How is the press playing this? Will the vote come back to haunt them later? Do they owe any favors—vote trades—to other legislators? More often than not, a legislator who's wishy-washy on a bill will trade his vote with a second legislator who does care about that bill, so that the first legislator can receive a favor the next time. Use politics: Coax legislators into coaxing their colleagues to vote yes on nonsmokers' rights. You will have to craft this vote as one that must stand on its own merits, one that legislators will have to justify on election day.

If your GASP's budget is large enough, buy newspaper, radio, or television advertising time urging people to contact their legislator in support of the bill, and urging legislators to vote for it. Even a bare "tombstone" advertisement explaining the benefits of the law and countering tobacco's rhetoric about it can go a long way toward winning the minds of legislators.

Particularly articulate GASP members should be invited to schedule visits with their own legislators. After all, the job of a representative is to listen to his electorate. As the vote draws close, your group's leaders and celebrities should arrange another formal meeting with the most important swing votes.

Plan to testify at hearings. Some legislators are persuaded by what they learn at hearings, others hardly ever attend; still others are there in body, but have developed the ability to nap with their eyes open. Nevertheless, hearings are important. The media often pay attention to them, and legislators are just as likely to be persuaded by what television or newspapers say about a hearing as what they hear themselves. Representatives who are converted nonsmokers' rights advocates may encourage other legislators to vote for the legislation. It's essential, therefore, that you testify at these hearings. And as an important player in the local nonsmokers' rights movement, you should be invited to testify. Usually, "being invited" means calling or writing the committee's chair and asking to testify: Be sure to do this well before the time allotted for testimony is booked. It's also important that many different pro-nonsmokers' rights legislation spokespeople testify. Possible spokespeople include a physician, insurance-company executive, fire-department officer, representative of the local chapter of the American Cancer Society, PTA member, and, of course, your celebrities. *Make sure your spokespeople are articulate and can speak on their feet:* Legislators are going to ask *tough* questions, so everyone who testifies should be prepared. Some lawmakers will be hostile and will have been prepped by the Tobacco Institute—their questions can be nasty. Your testifiers must be able to talk about all aspects of passive smoking and why this legislation is the solution. When witnesses can't express their views clearly, legislators take that as a sign that there are weaknesses with the bill that person is supporting.

Occupy as much time as possible at these hearings. The Tobacco Institute probably won't testify, but they will send their allies: restaurant and hotel associations, paid scientists, attorneys, and civic leaders. Anticipate what pro-tobacco people will say, and rebut their perspectives during your testimony (in addition to stressing the many positive reasons for nonsmokers' rights laws). Try to coordinate your side's testimony; cover all the subjects, but avoid duplication and dullness. Each witness should focus on his own speciality: physicians on health, insurance representatives on health and costs, PTA members on smoking's effects on children, and so forth.

Offer to write questions that friendly and undecided committee members can ask witnesses. Because you're more familiar with the issue, you can prepare better questions than legislators can, and because committee members and their staffs are busy, they may accept your offer. Prepare different questions for each legislator, and, make the questions specific to each witness. Here are some sample questions:

To Hotel and Restaurant Association Spokespeople:

- In Fairfax County, Virginia; Palo Alto and Beverly Hills, California; and Nassau County, New York, restrictions on smoking in restaurants hasn't hurt business at all. In fact, there's frequently a wait for tables. Why do you think this city would be any different?
- If you say that "if the marketplace demanded no-smoking sections, restaurants would provide them," how do you account for the Gallup survey that says 77 percent of the adult population wants separate smoking and no-smoking areas?
- How many members of your association have no-smoking sections? Do you know how these no-smoking sections have worked?

To Attorneys:

- Have you looked at the evidence from San Francisco, Los Angeles, San Diego, and Minnesota regarding enforcement costs and problems? Those cities and state have had no major or minor difficulties implementing their nonsmokers' rights laws.

- Why do you say that a nonsmokers' rights bill would turn ordinary citizens into law breakers? What evidence do you have for that? Do you think our citizens are so anti-law?

To Tobacco Institute Representatives (Should They Testify):

- Do you think that mainstream smoking causes disease?
- Do you know how a flu virus infects the body or how a jet engine works? [They'll have to say "no."] But you accept the facts—that being coughed at by someone with the flu isn't a good idea, and that the TWA plane you're going to take back to Washington will work. Even if you don't know the precise mechanism by which they work. Is all knowledge predicated on fully knowing the way in which things operate?
- What evidence would be necessary for you to conclude that passive smoking can be dangerous, since you don't seem to accept the conclusions of the Surgeon General or National Academy of Sciences?
- How much are you spending on lobbying here?
- What local organizations are you funding?
- How did you estimate the costs for implementing our nonsmokers' rights laws? Why do you think the costs for enforcing nonsmokers' rights laws in other cities are so low?
- Do you think that serious public health issues should be resolved by common courtesy?

To Scientists:

- Do you or have you ever received funding from any tobacco organizations?
- Have you read the Surgeon General's report on passive smoking? Do you think the Surgeon General is wrong?

- On public health concerns shouldn't we err on the side of caution?

As the day of the vote approaches, check that all the legislators you rated number 1 to make sure they are going to be there. If any pro-nonsmokers' rights representatives are going to be away, coax them into rearranging their schedules or get them to give their proxy to another clean-air supporter. Count the votes before: If it looks close, inform those legislators who plan to be absent that it's going to be a tight vote and that the nonsmokers' rights legislation could lose because of their one vote! Use any clout you have—celebrities, the bill's sponsors, press attention—to ensure that your supporters are there when heads are counted. Lots of votes are won and lost because of absences.

Tobacco's Lobbying Tactics

Lobbying council members and legislators isn't your only concern; you'll have to be prepared to combat the cigarette industry's campaigns.

Depending on how large an area the nonsmokers' rights legislation you've proposed would affect, you can expect a forceful tobacco presence. Sometimes tobacco's activities will be overt, but when they're more subtle, your job will be letting everyone—the press, legislators, and ordinary citizens—know about what they're up to.

As mentioned earlier, the Tobacco Institute will form a citizens' group called something like Citizens for Common Sense. The group will not be a grass-roots organization; instead it will be formed from the top down. The Tobacco Institute will hire a campaign manager to run a cigarette-industry-funded group.

Start with revealing the emperor's nakedness: Just about all of the spokespeople on the side of tobacco are paid; many may be from out of town. Some of the people testifying against the nonsmokers' rights legislation, appearing in television interviews, or quietly lobbying legislators, are paid public relations consultants and attorneys—hired hands in more honest vernacular. Be on the watch for former prominent officials who advocate no restrictions on smoking; chances are extremely good that they are remunerated by the Tobacco Institute. You may have to do some digging to uncover the names of the individuals and firms who are being paid by the Tobacco Institute.

The pro-nonsmokers' rights side, in contrast, is comprised of volunteers who live and work in the area. Doctors, lawyers, secretaries, blue collar, white collar workers—regular folks. It's important that the appearance of this campaign converges with its reality—average Joes and Janes versus the tobacco industry. Because as long as it doesn't, the Tobacco Institute will continue to wield its powers of deception.

The tobacco industry is large. Tobacco companies don't just produce cigarettes, but manufacture a host of friendly products, as well. Philip Morris owns Miller Beer and 7-Up; R.J. Reynolds is RJR Nabisco and owns Kentucky Fried Chicken, Del Monte, Hawaiian Punch, Heublein, and Harvey's Bristol Cream; Brown & Williamson Tobacco owns Saks Fifth Avenue, People's Drug, and Hardee's Restaurants; American Tobacco owns Franklin Life Insurance, Sunshine Biscuits, and Master Lock; the Liggett Group owns Carlsberg Beer, Alpo pet food, and Intercontinental Hotels; Lorillard owns CNA Financial, Loews Theaters, and Bulova Watch. The tobacco industry uses its clout through these subsidiaries. They may use executives from their subsidiaries to lobby, or they may use their influence to prevent GASP from having access to the media. Tony Schwartz, a media expert in New York, has documented that some radio stations are unwilling to air antismoking commercials because they are afraid that the cigarette companies will withdraw advertising of their nontobacco products. In 1983, when the San Francisco Board of Supervisors was considering nonsmokers' rights legislation, Del Monte, a subsidiary of R.J. Reynolds, lobbied heavily against the bill.

The industry will use its store-bought clout to lobby legislators. When you visit your representatives, ask them whether any antilegislation people have been around. Talk with the legislator about how that lobbyist is an employee of the cigarette industry, and how you are concerned that in this battle between the people and tobacco dollars, the majority's voice is not being heard. Hopefully, the legislator will assure you that the nonsmokers' rights views are being heard.

Rhetoric is the Tobacco Institute's second best weapon; they have become pretty practiced at presenting their standard arguments in public forums and in literature. They will use isolated examples to "prove" their generalities. For example, to show that nonsmokers' rights laws are capricious and draconian, they may dredge up an instance where someone was tried for violating these laws; to show that nonsmoking sections in restaurants are a bad idea, the Tobacco Institute will find a restaurant or two in which there's a line for the smoking section. And so on. The examples they cite are rarities, *and* often the Tobacco Institute doesn't present all the information about a particular circumstance; they're not interested in revealing the *whole* truth. The themes used to sway legislators include:

- There's no proof that environmental tobacco smoke is harmful. Annoyances, like fingernail tapping and smoking, don't require legislation.
- The environmental tobacco smoke health issue is still a subject of debate. We support continuing research to resolve questions about smoking and health.
- Laws shouldn't be used when common courtesy works well.
- Nonsmokers' rights legislation will be costly for the state to implement.
- The law promotes one-man tyranny in the workplace, because a single nonsmoker can dictate smoking policy to an entire office.
- Valuable police time and court time will be usurped by these laws.
- Antismoking laws are difficult to enforce.
- Antismoking laws will pit smoker against nonsmoker.
- Antismoking regulations will be expensive to employers.
- No-smoking sections in restaurants will drive away patrons.
- The marketplace should determine whether no-smoking sections are needed.
- Nonsmokers' rights laws are unconstitutional.
- Antismoking laws deprive smokers of their rights to smoke.

The Tobacco Institute will try to confuse voters and legislators about smoking. They'll point to the "inconsistent" evidence about the health effects of involuntary smoking. They'll create concern in voters' minds about the possible costs and civil liberties implications of enacting these laws. And they will try to raise doubts about the necessity of nonsmokers' rights legislation. This is a practical and dangerous campaign strategy: Voters and legislators who are confused about a referendum tend to vote no, and that's the tobacco position.

Expect a propaganda blitz as the vote draws closer. The tobacco lobby may choose to send each legislator a letter signed by a celebrity they've *hired*, they may purchase a full-page advertisement in the newspaper, they may have one of their political supporters on the day of the vote offer a compromise bill that's no compromise. Whatever they do, the Tobacco Institute won't relax toward the end of the campaign. Be prepared to contact every legislator, warning them that the substitute bill is not acceptable; be prepared to hand-deliver press releases countering the Tobacco Institute's fallacious claims; be prepared to send special-delivery letters to council members. Be prepared for anything.

Anything includes failure. You're up against terribly strong competition. In politics, money does talk, so you shouldn't be disappointed if you lose on the first round. It took Californians for Nonsmokers' Rights (now called Americans for Nonsmokers' Rights) two times to get the nation's strictest workplace smoking laws passed. Seasoned politicians will tell you that, frequently, good legislation doesn't succeed the first, second, or even third time. But once enacted, no nonsmokers' rights laws have ever been repealed—though the tobacco industry has tried. Sometimes the first effort warms legislators to the idea of nonsmokers' rights. If your bill does not pass, prepare to introduce it again next year. Next year, the Tobacco Institute will have more legislative battles with which to contend, spreading its resources even thinner. And you'll have gained experience, new members, and more money. In the meanwhile, continue to educate people about nonsmokers' rights, encourage businesses and restaurants to respect the rights of nonsmokers, get to know legislators socially. Perhaps develop a handbook for businesses on why and how to create a smokefree workplace. Write op-ed articles. Your GASP might even consider forming a political action committee (PAC) to raise money for council members who voted in favor of your bill.

The Next Steps

GASP should monitor the legislation once it's in place. Although nonsmokers' rights laws are primarily self-enforcing, there will be an occasional problem. Your group can serve as an informal mediator when these problems occur; it can educate businesses about the law and offer to answer questions. Keep track of any problems that do occur. The Tobacco Institute will be watching the progress of this law as well, and they won't hesitate to exaggerate any minor problem and develop a propaganda data base for the next legislative campaign. You'll need to be able to defend against the cigarette industry's attempts to turn isolated instances into "I told you sos." On a more active level, you might also consider offering No Smoking signs for free or for a nominal cost, as well as booklets about passive smoking, health, and the law. After a year, you'll discover that the law has cost very little to enforce, taken little of the city or state's time, and generally made everyone happy. In fact, you will find that the nonsmokers' rights regulations have been so popular that it's time to introduce even more pro-clean-air regulations or, if you were working at the city level, to campaign for county or statewide regulations.

And what about the future? In the late 1980s a huge campaign, the Media-Advertising Partnership for a Drug-Free America, was launched. It aimed at getting youth to "just say no" to marijuana, cocaine, PCPs, crack, and heroin. It ignored tobacco, even though "tobacco use is one of the most important pathways to marijuana use among adolescents."[2] That's wrong. If we believe that it's wrong for teenagers to do drugs, then a national antidrug campaign ought to include tobacco. About 90 percent of all smokers start before they are nineteen years old. The future of nonsmokers' rights rests with our children. If they choose not to smoke, then ten or twenty years from now there won't be any problem with no-smoking sections because there won't be any smokers.

NOTES

(1) *Cleveland Plain Dealer,* April 6, 1986, p. P31.
(2) *New Jersey Medicine,* February 1988, p. 103.

CHAPTER 6

No Smoking in the Workplace

A patient with tuberculosis has the right to cough, but not in anyone else's face.

Dr. Peter Morgan,
Scientific Editor,
Canadian Medical Association Journal

Workplace Smoking Restrictions Are Like Health and Safety Regulations

The workplace has improved dramatically since the beginning of the industrial revolution. Starting with child labor protection laws and progressing to the complex web of statutes that regulate everything from exposure to individual chemicals to workers' compensation, a virtual battalion of laws has been enacted to protect workers from dangerous working environments.

Progress toward health and safety in the workplace has been slow; at times corporations have resisted laws that require them to install safety equipment, and opposed laws that prohibit certain profitable labor practices. At other times, headway toward a safer and healthier workplace has been hampered by myopia—the government and employers frequently did not recognize particular substances or practices as dangerous. For example, workers painted radium on old-style glow-in-the-dark watches. In between paint strokes, the watch dial painters licked the brushes to coax the bristles into cooperating. In those days, nobody knew that radium caused cancer, but many of these workers, mostly women, died from horrible cases of mouth cancer. The link was only made years later. A similar story can be told for asbestos. Though asbestos is a magnificent material for insulation and fire resistance, in the early days nobody understood that it caused mesothelioma—an almost always fatal cancer of the tissues surrounding the lungs. And only in the last dozen years has wearing ear protectors been recognized as a way of preventing hearing loss among people who work with heavy industrial equipment.

Smoking in the workplace is going through a similar process, because only recently have we become certain that inhaling other people's smoke is dangerous. People spend a lot of time at work—a third of the day, and about a quarter of their adult lives. Air contaminated by cigarette smoke is now known to produce burning eyes, allergic reactions, lung cancer, emphysema, heart disease, headaches, fetal damage, and a host of other disorders. Just a few cigarettes can make the air unhealthy for an entire office.

There's an interesting difference between most labor laws and the nascent workplace smoking restrictions. Unlike other health and safety regulations that are promulgated by the federal or state governments, workplace smoking restrictions are usually initiated by the employer or the employees. And business-inspired workplace smoking restrictions are usually more stringent than state laws. This change—from government-inspired health regulations, to businesses taking the initiative—has come about for several reasons.

First, over the past century, employers, thanks to congressional, executive, and judicial promptings, have developed a sense of responsibility for their employees' health. This enlightened philosophy hasn't spread throughout corporate America, but many businesses believe that ensuring their workers' health is the right thing to do.

Second, modern equipment such as computers, electronic switching equipment, and heavy machinery can be harmed by cigarette smoke. The particulates contained in sidestream cigarette smoke can reduce the lifetime of machinery and electronic equipment or cause it to malfunction. *Even Philip Morris does not permit smoking around the equipment used to manufacture 150 million cigarettes a day.*

The third—the bottom-line reason—is that companies have discovered that a no-smoking or restricted-smoking policy saves the company money. A lot of money.

- Insurance rates drop when people don't smoke at work, partly because smokers are healthier, but also because the fire rates are reduced when there are no matches, lighters, and smoldering cigarettes around.

- Moreover, smokers are involved in twice as many job-related accidents as nonsmokers.[1]

- Maintenance costs drop dramatically when there are no ashtrays to clean, no ashes ground into carpets, and no curtains and carpets to de-smoke. Employees in nonsmoking environments also have lower dry-cleaning bills because their clothes don't get odoriferous as often.

- Absenteeism also declines—cigarette smokers are out sick up to 45 percent more often than nonsmokers.[2] Smokers are 50 percent more likely to be hospitalized than nonsmokers. Smoking can lower a person's intellectual faculties because the carbon dioxide in cigarette smoke reduces the amount of oxygen reaching the brain. Smoking breaks cost the company productivity. All told, each smoker costs her employer about $350 per year in short-term costs. When you consider long-term effects spanning ten to fifteen years, such as premature death and disability, *each smoker costs her employer over $1,000 per year!* And nonsmokers who are exposed to tobacco smoke in the workplace also cost employers approximately $50 per nonsmoker a year, mostly through increased illness. Smoking—on and off work—costs the United States about $53 billion in lost productivity annually.

- Smoking costs each employee $27,000 over a lifetime in lost wages and cigarette costs.

- *The final bill for the country for all smoking-related costs including lost wages and medical care is over $64 billion a year.*

Twenty-one percent of companies with nonsmoking policies initiated their restrictions in response to employee pressure, but over 18 percent developed their programs because management believed that smoking is harmful to employee health, according to a 1986 survey by Donald Peterson and Douglas Massengill.[3] Another 8.7 percent of companies surveyed thought their nonsmoking policies would reduce insurance or other health costs.

A survey by Robert Half International found that when having to choose between equally qualified smokers and nonsmokers, personnel decision-makers picked nonsmokers by a fifteen-to-one ratio.

No smoking in the workplace is now in the mainstream of American business thought. It's respectable and intelligent to prohibit smoking in the workplace. Fifty-four percent of American businesses have some kind of no-smoking policy; between 2 and 6 percent of U.S. companies ban smoking altogether or restrict it to designated smoking rooms and only during work breaks. Almost 2 percent of businesses hire only nonsmokers. Many companies have programs to help their employees quit smoking, and 5 percent of U.S. employers offer monetary gifts to workers who quit!

And no smoking in the workplace is growing fast. In 1986, 36 percent of U.S. companies had smoking policies; in 1987, it was 54 percent! In 1986, 6 percent of American companies banned smoking in all corporate offices; in 1987, that figure had doubled to 12 percent![4]

How respectable are nonsmoking policies at work? Here are some of the companies chosen at random that have formal workplace smoking restrictions:

Boeing Company
Pacific Northwest Bell
Connecticut Mutual Life Insurance Company
Control Data Corporation
General Motors
Ford
Texas Instruments
Aetna Life and Casualty
Campbell Soup
Stride Rite Corporation
Levi Strauss
Bank of America
Merck and Company
Hewlett-Packard
IBM
Procter and Gamble
L.L. Bean
U.S. Army
U.S. Air Force

U.S. General Services Administration (the boss for a million
federal workers, including all military and civilian employees
at the Pentagon)

Only the Tobacco Institute and its accomplices regard nonsmokers'
rights legislation as something inspired by "fanatics" or as the
"tyranny of the minority."

As might be expected, the industry with the greatest proportion of
workplace smoking restrictions is the health care industry—over 92
percent have a policy on smoking. The industry with the second
highest percentage of no-smoking regulations is retail (82.6 percent),
then finance (61.4 percent), manufacturing (57.2 percent), transportation (50 percent), service (48.6 percent), and insurance (18.2 percent).

Employers have found that nonsmoking policies live up to the
employers' expectations in reducing costs and increasing productivity.
But they also find that nonsmoking policies are easy to implement. One
of the reasons for this is the overwhelming support for smoking
restrictions. *A 1987 Gallup poll conducted for the American Lung
Association discovered that 86 percent of nonsmokers, 64 percent of
current smokers, and 76 percent of former smokers believe that there
should be separate smoking and nonsmoking areas at work or that
smoking should be banned entirely.*

In June 1985, Pacific Bell completely banned smoking. Not a single
employee of Pacific Bell's fifteen thousand workforce quit as a result
of this policy. But, 25 percent of the company's smokers signed up for
a program to stop smoking, and employees who remained smokers cut
back the number of cigarettes they smoke a day by 31 percent. (More
examples of successful workplace smoking policies are described later
in this chapter.)

It's when businesses do not have workplace smoking restrictions
that problems arise. Nonsmokers who complain about tobacco frequently find, much to their dismay, that common courtesy is just a
poetic alliteration. According to Myra Romans, executive director of
Fresh Air for Nonsmokers in Washington state and an employee of
Group Health Cooperative (the first company in Washington state to
completely ban smoking), nonsmokers who request no-smoking areas
are "flamboyantly ignored. They are being treated as trouble-makers.
They call us and they say, 'What can we do to improve the situation

in our workplace?' '' The solution to this dilemma is not to rely on common courtesy, because it is not common at all, but to institute workplace smoking restrictions for everybody.

Most people—smokers and nonsmokers—recognize that smoking is dangerous. Workplace smoking restrictions and smoking-cessation programs can go a long way toward increasing a worker's overall health and a company's fiscal health. But a well-implemented program can do more: It can boost morale by showing that the company cares about its workers. Many companies restrict smoking around sensitive machinery—smoking restrictions show that a firm holds the health of its equipment and workers in equal regard. Smoking regulations foster an image of corporate concern, where everybody is important to the firm.

A safe workplace—free from cigarette smoke—is a right, not a luxury. When pursuing workplace smoking restrictions keep in mind that curtailing smoking at work will protect your health, and you should be bold and persistent about pursuing a nonsmoking policy at work.

INITIATING A NO-SMOKING POLICY AT WORK

Find Out About Your Company's Current Smoking Policy

The first step toward a smokefree workplace is finding out whether your company has or is considering a policy on restricting smoking. If you're lucky, your firm will be one of the 21 percent of U.S. companies that are considering a nonsmoking policy, in addition to the 54 percent that already have some policy, and so the hardest work will already be done—convincing management to begin thinking about the problem.

Some companies have policies that restrict smoking in a few places such as corridors, open spaces, around valuable electronic equipment and machinery, but not in enough areas to protect all the company's workers from tobacco fumes. You need to know the status of your firm's smoking policy before you pursue a more restrictive—and healthier—program. Check whether your company's policy is formally written down, or simply a custom.

Take an Informal Survey of People in Your Company

Talk with your coworkers about nonsmoking. Find out who else has been silently fuming every time they breathe smoke. At this stage you will want to accomplish three objectives: 1) Learn how your coworkers feel about smoking at work, 2) get a sense for who's behind you, and who will oppose nonsmoking policies, and 3) help people to start thinking about restricting smoking so that their minds will become even more receptive to the idea later.

At this stage, don't be confrontational; just be curious. Start a file system which groups people into three categories: 1) in favor of restricting smoking, 2) against workplace smoking restrictions, 3) undecided. Jot down what your coworkers have to say about nonsmokers' health regulations. Talk informally with as many people in as many different departments as you can including management, clerical, support, blue collar, and professional. You may be surprised to discover that some smokers support limiting or banning tobacco at the office.

Educate Yourself About Nonsmoking in the Workplace

This is crucial for waging a successful campaign for nonsmokers' rights, and it is doubly essential before you begin the next phase of action, talking with management about putting together smoking restrictions. Even if the majority of people in your firm support nonsmokers' rights (and unless you are in the tobacco business, they will), there will always be some who need to be convinced about the health effects of tobacco and the benefits of restricting smoking. "Don't rock the boat," and "if it ain't broke, don't fix it" mentalities exist at many businesses—you will have to explain why the absence of a smoking policy is, in fact, a smoking policy, and an unhealthy one. There are a lot of misconceptions about tobacco, health, and productivity you will have to dispel. And of course there may be a handful of individuals who vehemently oppose any change in smoking policy; you will have to reverse their opinions.

Health Effects

Passive smoking is clearly linked to heart disease, lung cancer, emphysema, and other disorders. It is one of several dangers that come under the rubric of indoor air pollution. An editorial in the respected *American Review of Respiratory Disease* (January 1986) said

> There is no disagreement about the biological plausibility of an association between passive smoking and lung cancer . . . Sidestream smoke has the same carcinogens and cocarcinogens as mainstream smoke, most at significantly increased concentrations . . .

Being around cigarette smoke all day long can produce disease. The Replace and Lowrey study which appeared in *Environmental International* in 1985 estimated that between five hundred and five thousand lung-cancer deaths a year are caused by involuntary smoking. And the Office of Technology Assessment in its conservative 1986 report, *Passive Smoking in the Workplace: Selected Issues* concluded:

> Examined together, the evidence is generally consistent with an increased risk of lung cancer, on the order of a doubling of risk, among nonsmokers regularly exposed to environmental cigarette smoke compared with nonsmokers without exposure . . . The data are sufficient to warrant serious concern . . .
> There is evidence that environmental tobacco smoke is an acute respiratory irritant in healthy adults.

James Replace, a scientist at the Environmental Protection Agency, further estimates that the lung cancer risk for nonsmokers in the workplace is "250 to 1,000 times the level of acceptable risk using standard federal guidelines for carcinogens in air or water or food" depending on how good, or poor, a building's ventilation is.[5] That should be enough incentive.

Lung cancer is not the only danger from involuntary smoking in the workplace. No matter how healthy you are, your lungs, your heart, and your circulatory system can be affected by breathing secondhand smoke—enough to damage your health. Studies have shown that the lungs of nonsmokers who work in smoky offices for years resemble the lungs of smokers—they are blackened and in a predisease condition. For people with any kind of lung or heart problems, exposure to smoke in the workplace may seriously exacerbate these conditions.

Passive cigarette smoke is as toxic as smoke which is directly inhaled. Sidestream smoke contains significant quantities of DMNA (dimethylnitrosamine), which produces cancer in all animal species and which can produce cancer after both multiple and single exposures. Sidestream smoke also contains benzopyrene, 2-naphthylamine, and 4-aminobiphenyl—three established, potent carcinogens. What exactly are these strange-sounding chemicals? They are substances for which "no exposure or contact by any route—respiratory, skin, or oral, as detected by the most sensitive methods—shall be permitted," according to the American Council of Government Industrial Hygienists. Sidestream smoke also contains carbon monoxide, which contributes to heart disease in the long run and reduces the ability of the blood cells to carry oxygen in the short term; cadmium, which destroys the fragile air sacs in the lungs and may promote emphysema; nicotine, which adversely affects the heart, making it pump faster; hydrogen cyanide, which damages the cilia in the lungs (cilia work like filter brushes to keep our lungs clean); radioactive elements such as polonium-210 which causes lung cancer, and over four thousand other chemicals and gasses.

A study by J.R. White and H.F. Froeb, reported in the *New England Journal of Medicine,* found that nonsmokers exposed to sidestream smoke in the workplace for long periods of time lost between 15 and 20 percent of their lung function.

Tobacco smoke has particularly pernicious effects on people who are allergic to any chemicals in sidestream smoke. But people with allergies are not the only ones bothered or harmed by involuntary smoking, though they may be the first to speak up. The problem is not with people who are medically allergic to cigarette smoke, the problem is with tobacco smoke—it harms everyone. Don't be misled by the false notion that the problem of smoking at work can be resolved by separating the few who have doctor's notes saying that they're allergic. People with allergies to cigarette smoke are akin to the canaries in the coal mine; they are the first harmed, but in a frighteningly short time, other people can start to show the effects.

In environments where workers are exposed to chemicals, smoking and this exposure can produce particularly dangerous synergisms. According to the Surgeon General:

> Chronic simple bronchitis has been associated with occupational exposures in both nonsmoking exposed workers and populations of exposed smokers in excess of rates predicted from the smoking habit alone . . .
>
> Asbestos exposure can increase the risk of developing lung cancer in both cigarette smokers and nonsmokers . . .
>
> Both tobacco smoke and some industrial pollutants contain substances capable of initiating and promoting cancer and damaging the airways and lung parenchyma. There is, therefore, an ample biologic basis for suspecting that important interactive effects between some workplace pollutants and tobacco smoke exist.[6]

Asbestos workers who smoke are ten times more likely to die prematurely than nonsmoking asbestos workers, and have a fifty- to ninety-times higher risk of developing lung cancer than someone who neither smokes nor works with asbestos. Uranium miners face a six-fold increased risk of lung cancer than their nonsmoking colleagues.

Most nonsmokers are unaware of the effects of involuntary smoking. But these effects are real—and very dangerous.

Ventilation

Smoking in the workplace is particularly dangerous because people spend a long time there—forty hours a week on average—and because the concentrations of tobacco smoke are usually very high. Office buildings are expensive places to heat and cool, so to keep the cool air in during the summer and the cold air out during the winter, modern buildings do not exchange indoor and outdoor air frequently. To lower costs, on average only 10 percent of the air inside an office building is recirculated from the outdoors in a given hour. Some buildings have almost no ventilation, and far too many don't have windows that open. As a result, tobacco smoke is constantly recirculated throughout office buildings; the more smokers, the more smoke accumulates.

Indoor air pollution is a more serious problem than outdoor air pollution. If the air outside were as smoky as the air is in a room with cigarette smokers, action would be taken immediately to clean it. If the air outside contained the same dangerous and potentially deadly gasses and particles as does the air in an office with several smokers, the government would be forced to do something about it right away.

Most of the time, tobacco smoke is invisible to the nose and eye. But just because you can't smell tobacco smoke, doesn't mean that the air is safe. A good proportion of the four thousand-plus chemicals in cigarette smoke, including carbon monoxide and polonium-210, are odorless, colorless, and tasteless, but still dangerous. It takes the ventilation system in a typical building three hours to rid the air of smoke from a single cigarette, assuming that there are no new cigarettes lit. With two or more smokers smoking just a cigarette an hour, the atmosphere in an office has ever-increasing amounts of tobacco smoke in it. According to one report:

> Under the practical range of ventilation conditions and building occupation densities, the respirable particle levels generated by smokers under typical conditions overwhelm the effects of ventilation even when applicable standards are observed.[7]

How high are the concentrations of tobacco smoke? *An average worker in an average office will inhale nicotine, tar, carbon monoxide, and other carcinogens and toxic materials at levels that are equivalent to smoking between two to three cigarettes each day!*

And if you are sitting close to a smoker (or more than one smoker), you will be inhaling even larger doses of tobacco smoke.

One popular method of separating smokers and nonsmokers at the workplace is to provide smoking lounges, where smokers can go to light up. Another alternative is to separate smokers and nonsmokers into different rooms. Although these are attractive-sounding ideas, and are better than forcing nonsmokers to work in the same area where cigarettes are being puffed, smoking lounges and segregation are not solutions. Because most ventilation systems are designed to circulate the air throughout a building, limiting smoking to only one or several locations fails. Smoke from a smoking lounge or from a private office quickly contaminates the air in the rest of the building. As people smoke in private offices or a smoking lounge during the day, the air throughout the building will grow steadily more contaminated. Walls provide virtually no barrier to tobacco smoke because *ventilation systems are designed to spread the air around evenly.*

The only safe smoking area is one that is not connected with the rest of the office's ventilation network. This is not as difficult or expensive to design as it appears. To create a smoking lounge, a particular room can be sealed off from the rest of the building's ventilation system; window air conditioners and interior heaters can be installed to regulate the temperature. However, to prevent the smoke-filled air from a smoking lounge from mixing with the rest of the building's air when the door to the lounge is opened, the air in that room must be constantly exchanged with outside air. The same is true for individual offices. Only offices with separate ventilation systems won't pollute the air in the rest of the building.

One idea that's offered as a solution is to install machines to clean the air. But technological solutions to the ventilation problem are always disappointing: Smokeless ashtrays are just a gimmick. Portable air cleaners are only marginally effective, because most cleaners remove only some tobacco smoke particles from the air. Gases, which comprise 90 percent of sidestream smoke and which contain such harmful compounds as carbon monoxide and hydrogen cyanide, are not affected by air cleaners. Neither are many of the smaller (.0002 to .01 microns) particulate constituents of tobacco smoke. These gases and small particles will reach nonsmokers' lungs even if air cleaners are used. Air cleaners are also expensive to buy, costing about $2,000 a room for one that will provide at least six air changes an hour, a rate that would not be effective with as few as four smokers in a room. An effective office air cleaner could cost $30,000. Ionizers, which purport to remove particles from the air through magnetic attraction, are ineffective against tobacco smoke. At best they will remove a handful of some of the larger particulates from secondhand smoke.

Smoke-filled air must be kept physically separate from the air that nonsmokers breathe. This is the only way of maintaining a smokefree office.

Productivity

Smoking on the job reduces the productivity of nonsmokers. The eye irritation, sore throats, headaches, coughing, nausea, allergy, and asthma attacks certainly don't help workers focus on their jobs. Because involuntary smoking also has major long-term effects, nonsmokers who breathe tobacco fumes may become chronically ill or die sooner than they would if they worked in a smokefree environment. Marvin M. Kristein, of the Department of Economics at the State University of New York at Stony Brook, estimates that "the minimal overall health status and performance damage to involuntary smokers is equal to one fifth of that for smokers of one pack per day plus."[8] This means that *nonsmokers exposed to cigarette smoke at the workplace cost their employers between $53 to $105 per person a year* in insurance and other costs. Looking just at health costs (factoring out cleaning, insurance, and other smoking expenses), workers who smoke involuntarily cost their employers between $26 and $56 annually. These figures do not include long-term health effects, and they don't include synergistic effects between involuntarily breathed tobacco smoke and other occupational hazards such as exposure to asbestos, petroleum fumes, industrial dust, ink gases, pesticides, and X rays. If you take into account the combined effects of passive smoking and these other pollutants, nonsmokers who are exposed to tobacco smoke at work may cost their employers between $104 and $486 a year.[9]

But the most significant losses in productivity come from smokers. Nationwide, smoking reduces the GNP by between $43 billion and $67 billion a year, and it costs American businesses from $13 to $47 billion each year. Why include this information in a book about *nonsmokers'* rights? Because a side benefit of workplace smoking restrictions is that such regulations encourage smokers to quit! Many workplace smoking restrictions are accompanied by quit-smoking programs. Thus, smokers, nonsmokers, and businesses *all* benefit from smoking restrictions.

Smokers have one of the highest rates of absenteeism of any group of workers. Eighty-one million work days are lost each year because of smoking-induced sickness.[10] Smokers are sick between 33 and 45 percent more often than nonsmokers, taking an average of two extra sick days per smoker annually (a low estimate), according to Professor Kristein.

In addition, smokers are 50 percent more likely to be involved in automobile accidents than nonsmokers[11] and two times more likely to become involved in accidents at work.

Kristein estimates that the average smoking employee costs her employer between $336 and $601 a year in short-term costs. Over a ten-year period, taking into account premature disability and death, each smoking employee costs his employer an average of $1,100 a year. Here's how he breaks down his estimate (January 1980 dollars):

Health	$204
Fire	$ 10
Workers' Compensation	$ 34
Life Insurance	$ 33
Absenteeism	$ 80
Productivity	$166
Involuntary Smoking	$105

Another analyst, William Weiss, a CPA and associate professor of business at Seattle University, estimates that each smoker costs his employer $4,611 a year. This difference comes about because Kristein's assumptions are conservative and include smokers taking only eight minutes a day to smoke, and smokers losing only two days a year due to smoking at a cost to the employer of $40 a day. In many instances, smokers spend more than eight minutes a day indulging their habit, are absent more than two extra days a year, and are worth more than $40 a day to their employer (this figure does not also include the cost of temporary employees). Kristein *does not* take into account damage to furniture and equipment, cleaning costs, and increased ventilation costs. Smokers account for 87 percent of the demand for ventilation in an office![12]

An article in the May 1981 issue of the British journal *Personnel Management* said that companies can save up to 10 percent in wages, 50 percent in furniture depreciation, 50 percent in cleaning costs, 30 percent in health insurance premiums, and 75 percent in disability benefits if they have a total no-smoking policy! Smokers at work don't just burn tobacco, they burn dollars, too.

Usually workplace smoking policies cost very little to implement. ⨍ Memos and signs, costing at most hundreds of dollars, are all a company needs to curtail smoking in the workplace. This cost is probably equal to the cost of replacing ashtrays. A program to induce employees to quit smoking costs more—between $100 to $200 an employee who wants to quit—but the savings in terms of reduced insurance, health care costs, and productivity are staggering.

A 1984 study conducted for Pacific Northwest Bell estimated that the lifetime cost of smoking for a forty-year-old who smokes two packs a day is $56,670. Another company estimated that for each smoking employee it coaxed into quitting, the company saved $73 in insurance costs a year.

AT&T, before divestiture, estimated that it lost 6 percent of its annual productivity because of employees who smoke—that came to $170 million a year! General Motors estimates that smoking-related costs add $500 to the price of every automobile.

At the U.S. Steel Corporation, researcher David Smith found that

> Employees who smoke have more work-loss days than those who have never smoked. In every age group, as the number of cigarettes per day in confirmed smokers increases, so also does sick absence. Male smokers of more than two packs per day have nearly twice as much absence as their nonsmoking associates; the heaviest women smokers of more than two packs a day miss more than twice as much time as their counterparts who do not smoke.[13]

Johnson & Johnson has cut absenteeism by 20 percent and hospitalizations by 30 percent through its no-smoking and quit-smoking policies. The savings have been three times the cost of implementing these programs.

When the Control Data Corporation discovered in 1980 that smoking employees had 25 percent higher health-care costs and 114 percent more hospital days than nonsmokers, it created a plan to coax workers into quitting. Employees are now not allowed to smoke, except in specifically designated areas, but are encouraged to participate in computer-assisted smoking cessation and wellness programs.

The Radar Electric Company in Seattle, Washington, has saved $125,000 a year since it banned smoking in 1977.

In 1977, the Merle Norman Cosmetics company in Los Angeles estimated that by banning smoking in offices, rest rooms, and in their factory, it saved $33,000 a year.[14]

In 1986, the American Contract Bridge League banned smoking in its tournaments.

On July 1, 1987, Mesa Partnership prohibited smoking in its corporate headquarters.

The Northern Trust Bank of Chicago has banned smoking for all of its 4,500 employees, except in lounges, and has created stop-smoking clinics.

The no-smoking rule at Lovejoy-Tiffany & Associates in Ann Arbor, Michigan, was instituted by the company's employees.

Even Deluxe Check Printing of Richmond, Virginia, *right next to Philip Morris*, has phased in a no-smoking policy (mandated by the company's main office in Minnesota). The policy included a quit-smoking program, and 40 percent of smokers did quit.[15]

Georgia Power Company bars smoking in all public areas, and, according to Gordon Van Mol, director of corporate communications, "now there's a real reluctance to light up anywhere."[16]

Fellows Manufacturing Company in Itasca, Illinois, banned smoking in December 1986. Company president James Fellows decided against separate lounges for smokers: "The rooms inevitably fill up with smoke no matter how much ventilation, and they can be expensive to build and operate." Fellows pointed out that his company's policy was successful because "we've been very careful to describe it as a clean-air policy, rather than a no-smoking policy."

Dow Chemical found that smoking workers in its Midland, Texas, facility were absent 5.5 days a year more than nonsmokers, costing the company $657,146 in excess wage costs alone. In addition, Dow found that smokers had three times the incidence of pneumonia, 41 percent more bronchitis and emphysema, a 200 percent greater incidence of circulatory problems, and 76 percent more respiratory diseases of all kinds. Smokers had 7.7 more disability days than nonsmokers, and during this three-and-a-half-year study, smokers died at a rate of 3.5 times more than nonsmokers.[17]

Workplace smoking restrictions help smokers cut back on the number of cigarettes they consume each day and help employers dramatically cut their costs. When combined with programs to help

smokers quit, companies, through nonsmoking policies, can save thousands or hundreds of thousands of dollars a year!

No Smoking in the Workplace Is 100 Percent American

Chapter 1 pointed out how much a part of the mainstream of American business thought workplace smoking restrictions are. A growing number of small and giant companies are initiating policies to reduce smoking, with the eventual goal of having a completely smokefree working environment. Curtailing, and especially, eliminating smoking at work is capitalistic and healthy—a rare, but powerful combination. An article in the *Harvard Business Review* asked, "Should an employer become involved in influencing the way employees spend their lives? . . . Is corporate involvement in health promotion appropriate?" The answer: "The answer is a resounding yes."[18]

Most employees support workplace no-smoking policies. According to the Bureau of National Affairs, 54 percent of companies with smoking restrictions said their employees supported these programs, 20 percent of employers said their workers had no significant reaction, just 10 percent reported opposition to workplace smoking limitations.[19] The longer workplace smoking restrictions are in place, the less opposition there is to them among employees. But always remember that while popular appeal is important to a program, good health is even more crucial, and that's what no-smoking policies are designed to promote—good health. Pacific Northwest Bell told its employees when it instituted its no-smoking policy, "There are a number of reasons why this decision was reached, but the major one is the health issues concerned with smoking." Initially, Pacific Bell had a "compromise" no-smoking policy, but changed that to no-smoking anywhere because, in the words of the company's director of human resources, "there was the problem of smokers who bordered nonsmoking districts. Their smoke would drift over."[20] Companies that have restrictions on smoking in the workplace have universally praised these policies. Only the tobacco companies think these policies don't work. (But how do they know? They don't have any no-smoking policies in their offices.)

Legal Issues

Companies have every legal right to initiate their own no-smoking policies. There are no laws and no judicial precedents which could constrain a company from completely banning smoking on its premises, or even from hiring only smokers if it wants. In fact, the converse is gaining legal ground; legislation, arbitration decisions, and court cases increasingly *require* businesses to protect the health of nonsmokers by providing no-smoking areas at work. Nearly two dozen states have laws curtailing smoking in private workplaces. Montana, for example, has a penalty of $500 or 90 days in jail for employers who don't comply with the state's no-smoking laws.

Remember, just because there are workplace smoking laws on the books, doesn't mean your company can't or shouldn't have its own policies. None of these laws say anything about programs to help people quit smoking. Your company can use your state or municipality's laws as a base on which to institute a comprehensive workplace smoking policy.

When labor and management go to binding arbitration over whether nonsmokers should be safe from cigarette smoke in the workplace, arbitrators side with the nonsmokers. In June 1985 the Federal Service Impasses Panel resolved a disagreement between the Department of the Army and Local 1920 of the AFL-CIO on smoking. The FSIP ruled in favor of the Army, which wanted strict prohibitions on where smokers could light up. In another 1985 dispute between the Department of Health and Human Services and Local 3937 of the AFL-CIO, the FSIP ruled in favor of HHS, concluding that "the prohibition against smoking in an open-space office, where employees have contacts with members of the public, will provide protection for both nonsmoking employees and clientele against health hazards associated with passive smoking. This kind of protection is especially important to the elderly and disabled persons who come to the District Office for assistance."

Arbitration is also standing behind employers who strictly enforce their smoking restrictions. In *Illinois Freedom Produce Corp. and Teamsters Local 722*,[21] independent arbitrator Ralph Novak ruled that Freedom Produce's no-smoking policy was reasonable and that the company could fire a delivery driver for smoking during an unauthorized break.

Employees are successfully suing their employers for nonsmoking work spaces. The most celebrated case occurred in 1976 involving Donna Shimp and her employer, New Jersey Bell. Shimp had worked for New Jersey Bell for fifteen years and had a good record at the company. Unfortunately, she was extremely allergic to tobacco smoke, and when she was transferred to an office in which seven of the thirteen employees smoked, Donna Shimp suffered. She initiated formal grievance proceedings, which culminated in an exhaust fan being installed in her office. The fan was ineffective. After complaining to the management some more, she was finally offered a lower position with lower pay in a smokefree office. Donna Shimp refused and sued. The New Jersey Superior Court ruled that employers have an obligation to provide safe environments for their workers, and employees have the *right* to work in a safe environment. The court said:

> It is clearly the law in this state that an employee has a right to work in a safe environment. An employer is under an affirmative duty to provide a work area that is free from unsafe conditions. . . . The evidence is clear and overwhelming. Cigarette smoke contaminates and pollutes the air, creating a health hazard not merely to the smoker but to all those around [the smoker] who must rely upon the same air supply.
>
> The right of an individual to risk his or her health does not include the right to jeopardize the health of those who must remain around him or her in order to properly perform the duties of their jobs.[22]

There's an amusing side to this case, too. New Jersey Bell didn't allow smoking around its switching equipment. The court again: "The rationale behind the rule is that the machines are extremely sensitive and can be damaged by the smoke. Human beings are also very sensitive and can be damaged by cigarette smoke."

No-smoking workplaces are a common-law right. Indeed, employers who do not provide clean air for nonsmokers are vulnerable to a law suit, as *Parodi* v. *Merit Systems Protection Board*[23] shows. Parodi, who was sensitive to cigarette smoke, sued her employer, the Merit Systems Protection Board, a government agency, to provide her with a smokefree workplace. Instead of doing that, the company encouraged her to retire early. They also denied Parodi disability income even though she had developed asthmatic bronchitis from exposure to sidestream smoke. The Court found that Parodi was not able to perform her job because she worked in a smoke-filled room, ruling that her employer, the federal government, must provide her with "suitable employment in a safe environment," meaning completely free of smoke, or pay her $500 a month until she reached retirement age. The Court also awarded Ms. Parodi retroactive disability payments of $20,000 because she had been unable to work since 1979.

Another interesting case, *Fuentes* v. *Workmen's Compensation Appeals Board,* created a legal precedent of holding employers responsible for an employee's illness if the employee smokes. The California Supreme Court ruled that an employer was liable for one-third of an employee's disability from emphysema because the employer permitted the worker "to inflict harm on himself" by smoking at work.

Helen McCarthy v. *State of Washington Department of Dental and Health Services*[24] provided another valuable precedent in favor of nonsmokers. The Washington State Supreme Court of Appeals ruled that a nonsmoker harmed by the smoking of her coworkers at work has the right to sue the employer for negligence. This decision paves the way for employees affected by involuntary smoking to sue their employers—not just to claim disability.

Iowa and California have taken an additional step toward awarding payments to workers. Nonsmoking workers who have to quit their jobs because 1) their coworkers smoke and 2) their employers won't provide no-smoking offices, are eligible for unemployment benefits. These kinds of decisions can adversely affect a company's pocketbook.

A California county employee, Ms. Batchelor, won a $17,500 suit against her employer.[25] Batchelor proved that she suffered from headaches, stuffiness, general flulike symptoms, and chronic nose bleeding because she had to work in a room with tobacco smoke.

In *Vickers* v. *Veterans Administration,*[26] a federal court in Seattle ruled that a worker could be considered handicapped and entitled to protection under the Rehabilitation Act of 1973 because he was sensitive to cigarette smoke. An airline flight-crew member won an award of $3,657.50 plus attorney's fees and all expenses because she had a severe allergic reaction to tobacco smoke while in flight.[27] Other workers, including bank tellers, clerical staff, and senior administrators, have sued and been awarded payments because their employers refused to provide them no-smoking areas in which to work. C&P

Telephone, which serves the Washington, D.C., Virginia, and Maryland region, reacted to being the target of a $110,000 suit for medical expenses related to smoking, by banning all smoking on the premises. C&P decided not to take any more chances.

Adin Goldberg, a partner with the New York law firm, Spengler, Carlson, Gubar, Brodsky and Frischiling, puts the legal issue in perspective: "In terms of limiting liability, setting a corporate policy is probably the best way to go now."

Managerial Benefits of a No-Smoking Policy

As long as your company has no policy on smoking there will be dissension between smokers and nonsmokers. Once the issue is raised, the problem will grow worse, "common courtesy" will crumble, and there will be even greater polarization between smokers and nonsmokers. Managers will have to spend increasing amounts of time refereeing smokers and nonsmokers and will have to make decisions without a formal policy to guide them. An approved policy restricting smoking in the workplace is the best way to resolve differences between smokers and nonsmokers.

STEPS TO GETTING A SMOKEFREE WORKPLACE

Talk with Management About Examining a No-Smoking Policy

The next step in the process toward a smokefree office is to ask management for permission to *study* the possibility of having workplace smoking restrictions. At this stage you are still not asking for any policy to be designed or decided on—you merely want management to give its blessing to an *examination* of the issue.

Present both pros and cons to management. Let your boss know that you and other employees are deeply concerned about, first your health, and second, your company's pocketbook. But, indicate that you also recognize that there may be employees who feel strongly about being allowed to smoke at work. Let management know that you know that any change in the status quo has to be handled gingerly. Explain that you intend to talk with smokers and nonsmokers, find out what your coworkers' concerns are, predict how workplace smoking restrictions would benefit or harm the company, how much they would cost to implement, what the best workplace smoking policy is for your company, and how other companies have fared with their workplace smoking limitations. Emphasize that restricting smoking in the workplace is not new, so there's a substantial amount of information available on how to develop a no-smoking policy.

Mention that Campbell Soup has had no-smoking at work since 1869!

In 1988 Allstate Insurance Company stopped smoking in all of its 5,800 buildings across the country.

Summarize in writing the information about the various issues involved with smoking at work, as well. Management likes paper, and presenting the health, structural, economic, legal, and ethical aspects of workplace smoking restrictions in memo form will give the bosses something to refer to as time goes on. It will also show that you are careful and serious. A memo will document the fact that you are following the proper procedure for obtaining limitations on smoking at work.

Talk to the most senior managers you can. They are the ones, after all, who will eventually have to decide on whether there should be a new policy and what form it should take. Lower-level management is usually squeamish about changing the status quo.

Use this opportunity to find out how your company's decision makers feel about no smoking at the office. Although your report should sound neutral in tone, you're actually subtly lobbying management at the same time. Try to see if you can discern changes in the attitude of management between the time when you first broach the subject and after you've presented your introductory report on the pros and cons of workplace smoking restrictions. Mention that you'd like to talk with other vice-presidents (or whomever) and find out their thoughts on this issue, too. Anticipate their concerns by saying that you will pay particular attention to how smokers feel about these ideas (though most smokers do support separate smoking and no-smoking areas). Tell management that you are aware that the union (if your company is unionized) will want to be involved in this process and that you plan to talk with them, too.

Focus on smoking, tobacco, health, and productivity. Avoid talking about smokers, because smokers aren't the problem; cigarette smoke is. The issue isn't lifestyle, so don't moralize.

Make especially clear that you are not even thinking about quickly instituting smoking restrictions. *Any change in policy, if one is accepted, will be gradually implemented.* It's important that your company's executives understand that limitations on smoking would come about in stages and be designed not to disrupt the company's operations.

You might want to mention that cigarette smoking is a drug problem, too. It's been classified as an addiction by the National Institute on Drug Abuse. *The Washington Post* reported, "So strong is the addiction that despite the risks of miscarriage or stillbirth, 70 to 80 percent of women who smoke continue to do so while they are pregnant."[28] Restricting or banning smoking can help your office attain a drugfree environment.

Remember, though, your main purpose at this stage is to obtain permission to form a committee to assess the viability of smoking restrictions. Once you have that permission, you can move on to the next step, forming a committee.

Keep a diary of all your activities. In addition, be a prolific correspondent with people in your firm. Write them thank-you letters, and if anyone promises you anything, confirm it in writing. It's helpful to have written documentation on your efforts to achieve a smokefree workplace.

Most important, retain your sense of humor and good nature throughout the campaign.

What to Do if the CEO or Vice-Presidents Are Adamantly Opposed to Workplace Smoking Restrictions

First, be careful, because it's easier to try to get workplace smoking restrictions while you have a job. Don't go ahead and organize without the permission of your company's president, unless your union says okay. If you employer still says NO!—you can still work through a union and be protected from reprisals. (More about unions later.) When the boss says, "No, no committee," unfortunately, that's the law. Except. Except, the head of your organization probably didn't hear or understand what you were saying about health and productivity. So let her hear it again. Nicely. Send a letter thanking the CEO for her time. Mention the reasons why you believe workplace smoking restrictions would save the organization money and attach a copy of the memo you originally included. Invite her to get in touch with you when she believes it would be appropriate to study the issue.

Meanwhile, continue to talk with your coworkers. Find out who is bothered by tobacco smoke. Ask those people to make appointments with their supervisors or with the CEO to discuss workplace smoking restrictions. The more people who ask for something, the greater the likelihood you will get it. You need to make an impression on the boss. And you will be able to, because over 80 percent of smokers, nonsmokers, and former smokers are behind workplace smoking restrictions.

Form a Committee to Evaluate Smoking Restrictions

Designate a head of the Tobacco Smoke Evaluation Committee (TSEC)—you are probably the best person for this. If a physician on staff or the president of your firm supports workplace smoking restrictions, designate him as committee head. You will end up doing the work, but it doesn't hurt to have someone with prestige or power behind you. From the onset, you and management should agree that management will make time to listen to the committee's recommendations, and ultimately evaluate them. Your committee should include *only* employees who support nonsmokers' rights, but it should include smokers. Later, when you design a policy, you'll want to get opinions from all employees, but for now your job is difficult enough without major disagreements among TSEC members. Get the committee to work as quickly as possible.

Continue your research on smoking and its effects on health and costs. This is a good time to get in touch with your local nonsmokers' rights organization and the national organizations involved with smoking and health. They will be able to provide you with moral support and valuable information.

Conduct formal interviews with as many people as possible in the organization. Include: the president, vice-presidents and department heads, supervisors or foremen, head of the medical department, safety and security chiefs, recreation or physical-education director, representatives from employee groups, and union representatives. Make sure you talk with at least one person from every category of employee who could be affected by workplace smoking limitations. Discuss:

- *How does smoking around the office affect people's productivity and health?* Who is experiencing eye irritation, headaches and sore throats? How do people feel about cigarette smoke around them?
- *Are employees aware of the health effects of smoking?* Do they know that the office's ventilation system carries smoke around the entire building and is detrimental even when they can't smell any tobacco?
- *Are there any pregnant women on staff?* Might there be any in the future? (Fetuses are especially harmed by secondhand smoke.)
- *Are executives aware of the economic and health costs of smoking?*
- *Where does smoke bother people most?* In their offices? In the cafeteria? The rest rooms? The hallways or elevators? Other common areas? How do people feel about attending meetings in smoke-filled rooms?
- *Has anyone ever complained about smoking before?*
- *How would workplace smoking restrictions affect the quality of life?* Would people feel healthier? Work harder?
- *What do employees think would be an ideal smoking policy?* The status quo? Limiting smoking to private offices only? Including a program to help get smokers to quit? Banning smoking entirely?
- *How many packs a day do smokers consume?* Are most smokers light users of tobacco or heavily addicted? Are there pipe or cigar smokers in the office?
- *Ask smokers: Would you be induced to quit if the company*

offered a stop-smoking program? Could you do so if the company paid for it or offered bonuses to people who didn't smoke?
- *What do you perceive as the potential problems with a no-smoking policy?*
- *What are the short- and long-term benefits of smoking restrictions?*

Circulating an anonymous questionnaire to every employee is another way to tabulate your coworkers' thoughts on smoking. If your company is small enough, or if the front office considers it worthwhile, a questionnaire can give you precise, numerical data on how many employees support a policy of no smoking in the workplace and what kind of policy they would like. Keep in mind, however, that people tend to embrace workplace smoking restrictions more fully *after* the policy is in place than while it's an abstraction. By asking coworkers their opinions about workplace smoking restrictions you open the door to their eventually accepting and supporting the concept.

Next, gather information that can help determine what shape the smoking restrictions should take. Examine:

- What are the current policies on smoking?
- What is the status of your office's and building's ventilation, heating, and air-conditioning system. How does air circulate through the building? How often is air recirculated? Are there any rooms with separate ventilation systems? Remember that in most offices only 10 percent of fresh air mixes with 90 percent of indoor air and tobacco smoke; a highly efficient, but rare, ventilation system will mix 20 percent outdoor air with 80 percent indoor air.
- Where are the rest rooms? Do people smoke there?
- Are there rooms in which there already is no smoking allowed because of sensitive equipment?
- Are there rooms which could be potential smoking lounges?
- What is the absenteeism rate among smokers versus non-smokers?
- What are the cleaning, equipment, and furniture-repair costs associated with smoking? Talk with the maintenance and

cleaning staff, because they will have a better feeling about
this than management.

- How does smoking affect your company's health, life and
  fire insurance rates?
- What role does the union play in determining workplace
  smoking restrictions? Does the contract with the union
  mention smoking? Is it a subject for mandatory negotiation?
  (Because smoking is a health issue, the employer has the
  right to take action to ensure the safety of his employees,
  even if the union wants to negotiate on this.)
- How are workmen's compensation costs structured?

Organize this information into three categories:

- Employee interests, concerns, and status, including infor-
  mation about smokers and nonsmokers.
- Structure of the physical plant.
- Ventilation system.

Decide on Specific Workplace Smoking Restrictions

You must enunciate specific goals for your business. No smoking
anywhere—the philosophies of Pacific Bell, Billy Graham Associates,
Johns-Manville (Denver and New Jersey), and the *Newport Daily
News* for example—is the best policy, and should always be your
objective even if it is not immediately attainable. There are two ways
to achieve a smokefree office.

First, smoking can be banned throughout the premises—the most
difficult objective unless senior management is behind you.

The second way is to limit smoking to a few designated smoking
areas *that have their own ventilation system,* and to encourage
employees not to smoke. Declare the workplace no smoking, except
where designated, such as smoking lounges and part of the cafeteria.
Cleaning bills and equipment replacement costs will be dramatically
reduced, as well. This option makes smoking a conscious decision,
and helps smokers cut back on the number of cigarettes they consume
each day. (And as fewer people smoke, costs drop still more!) Any
policy that sharply curtails—or bans—smoking leaves little doubt that

the company is committed to both improving its employees health and keeping costs down.

There are a large variety of possible policies from which to choose and a variety of ways to implement them. But regardless of the policy you adopt, workplace smoking restrictions should be implemented gradually. Keep in mind, too, that whatever path you think is most fitting to your situation, your objective should be to attain a smokefree environment. That means any workplace smoking policy should include helping smokers who want to quit.

Within the three major alternatives are many variations:

- Ban smoking entirely on the premises.
- Ban smoking indoors only.
- Prohibit smoking except for designated smoking areas (those with their own ventilation systems).
- Allow smoking breaks only during designated break times such as lunch and the morning coffee breaks.
- Provide smoking cessation programs.
- Provide monetary or other incentives to nonsmokers.
- Hire only nonsmokers.
- Remove cigarette vending machines.
- Permit smoking in private offices at all times.
- Permit smoking in private offices except when nonsmokers are present.
- Ban smoking at meetings.
- Permit smoking in any area that is made up of only smokers.
- Permit smoking unless someone objects. Let employees designate their own no-smoking areas.
- Have a comprehensive smoking education project.
- Have a separate no-smoking area in cafeterias and lounges (is ventilation adequate?).
- Install window air conditioners in rooms in which smoking is permitted.
- Ban smoking in areas with sensitive equipment and in libraries.
- Allow visitors to smoke only in reception areas.
- Don't allow visitors to smoke at all.
- Offer exercise classes.

Quit-Smoking Programs

As you can see, the possible combination of smoking policies is limitless. In addition, the policy can change over time toward workplace smoking restrictions.

A word about smoking-cessation programs is in order here. The most effective policies on workplace smoking include programs that encourage smokers to quit. For many companies, it may be *essential* that some inducements or assistance accompany the firm's smoking restrictions. Ninety percent of all smoking adults would like to quit if they easily could; 60 percent say they've tried and failed. Many, maybe most, of a company's smoking employees really want to quit smoking, to be healthier. But quitting is very, very difficult; nicotine is powerfully addictive. Persistence is the key ingredient for smokers who eventually quit; only 25 percent of smokers successfully stop smoking on the first try, but 73 percent quit by the fourth attempt.

A good smoking-cessation program offers information about smoking and the problems encountered by smokers who want to break away from this addictive poison. It talks about alternatives to smoking such as exercise, eating carrots, or drinking mineral water. Smoking-cessation programs use effective techniques to enable smokers to break their addiction—such as gradually weaning them off tobacco, rapid smoking, biofeedback, overeducation about the dangers of cigarettes, and hypnosis. Monetary and other awards can be used as incentives (remember, nonsmokers cost a company less than smokers).

Pioneer Plastics of Auburn, Maine, gave employees $25 to use at their favorite restaurant if they quit smoking; other firms provide nonsmokers and former smokers even more substantial bonuses such as discounts on life and health insurance. Intermatic, a manufacturer of heating equipment, allows employees to wager up to $100 that they can quit smoking. If they quit, they receive $100; if they lose, they donate $100 to the American Cancer Society. The Hartford Insurance company distributes carrot sticks and sugarless gum to help quitters, as well as reimbursing employees who successfully quit for the cost of the smoking-cessation program; they receive cash if they stay off cigarettes. At Hartford, smokers may take the program on company time. City Federal Savings and Loan Association of Birmingham, Alabama, has, since 1975, offered $20 a month to former smokers and to new, nonsmoking employees. Johnson & Johnson gives insurance discounts to employees who engage in four out of six "good health" practices that include wearing seat belts, weight control, exercise, and not smoking.

Small groups, individual counseling, reading material, weekly sessions, audio-visual demonstrations, and lectures may also be involved. A number of companies tie their smoking-cessation programs to the American Cancer Society's annual November Great American Smokeout. Bonne Bell in Lakewood, Ohio, also gives cash incentives along with its instructional programs to employees who quit. Bonne Bell combined its stop-smoking courses with other health-oriented programs—it's all part of the company's commitment to good health. (The company restricts smoking to only one room in the building and only during two fifteen-minute breaks or lunch.) At Bonne Bell, there's an awards program that gives $250 to employees who quit for six months; however, employees who join this program and resume smoking must pay the company $500! The money is donated to a voluntary association that promotes no-smoking programs. The Mahoning Culvert company of Canfield, Ohio, lets nonsmoking employees earn up to $1,500 over two years. Former smokers are asked to contribute 50 cents a day into a pool. If at the end of the year, the employee still doesn't smoke, the company will add $817.50 to the pool, giving the total $1,000 to the ex-smoker. During the second year, former smokers can earn another $500 the same way.

Wellness programs that include both assistance in quitting smoking and programs in exercise, nutrition, alcohol and drug abuse, and psychological support can go a long way toward improving the overall health of a company's employees.

Writing Your Workplace Smoking Policy

Your policy statement should have nine parts:

A SIMPLE STATEMENT OF OBJECTIVES. In a couple of short sentences you should describe what you want to accomplish, and mention that the company has concluded that tobacco smoke is harmful to both nonsmokers and to the economic well-being of the firm.

THE OFFICIAL POLICY STATEMENT. The precise wording, by management, of what the business' new workplace smoking restrictions will be. The wording should be clear and direct, and should include the date the policy starts. Be sure to say whether a quit-smoking plan is included in the policy. Mention the specifics of when and where smoking breaks can be taken.

TIMETABLE FOR IMPLEMENTATION OF THE POLICY. Any policy, especially one which ultimately bans smoking, should proceed gradually. This gives smokers a chance to decide whether they want to quit and how they are going to quit. Workplace smoking restrictions are most easily implemented in stages, starting with educating employees about the policy and culminating with your objective. Larger businesses generally need more time to implement workplace smoking restrictions.

REASONS FOR WORKPLACE SMOKING RESTRICTIONS. This section should elaborate on the health and economic impacts of smoking. Include information about air circulation. You should explain why the particular policy you've chosen was selected over others. Sell the policy here—why will it benefit all employees? Discuss trends in workplace smoking restrictions, and your company's attitude toward the health of its employees.

WHO THE POLICY APPLIES TO. Ideally, workplace smoking restrictions should apply to everyone—or at least everyone who shares the common ventilation system. People shouldn't be excluded just because they have a private office; but if you do exempt private offices, prohibit smoking while nonsmokers are present. Keep exceptions to a minimum and don't forget visitors! Workplace smoking restrictions work best when they apply to everyone across the board.

RESPONSIBILITY FOR IMPLEMENTATION. Which person or department is in charge of implementing, monitoring, and enforcing the policy? Point out that this department will also educate employees about smoking and health, as well as about this policy. *Communication is probably the most crucial element of workplace smoking restrictions:* smoking employees will only be comfortable if they understand the policy, understand its rationale, and know who they can go to for answers. Explain how the policy will be enforced and what the penalties are for smoking. It's helpful to organize an open meeting between smokers and senior management, so employees can express their concerns and management can reassure smokers that the policy will be fair and supportive. In any case, both smokers and nonsmokers should know to whom people should complain when they have a problem.

SMOKING CESSATION PROGRAMS. Explain your company's plan to help smokers quit. Mention that it is voluntary, but don't forget to point out any incentives the plan includes.

MECHANICS. Will no-smoking areas be marked with no-smoking signs? Are cigarette vending machines going to be removed? Will ashtrays be placed at the outskirts of no-smoking areas?

RELATED POLICIES. Will the company be hiring only nonsmokers from now on? Will nonsmokers be given a break in insurance or additional medical benefits? (Will the company be switching to an insurance firm that offers discounted policies to nonsmokers?) Will the company be adding physical education or wellness programs?

Working with Unions

Unions are in a pickle when it comes to smoking because they represent smokers and nonsmokers. Whichever position the union takes on smoking in the workplace, it will alienate some of its members; and there are plenty of other issues it can pursue that won't estrange any constituents. Unions are also worried that an emphasis on passive smoking may draw attention away from other serious workplace health issues such as asbestos and petrochemicals. When the Surgeon General issued his report highlighting a dangerous synergism between tobacco smoke and other health hazards in the workplace, the AFL-CIO issued a strong rebuttal. (The Surgeon General said afterward that this 1985 report, *The Health Consequences of Smoking,* should not and did not detract from the importance of these other serious health problems.) There may be times when the management is behind workplace smoking restrictions, but the union isn't. In these cases you need to coax your shop steward and other union leaders into helping you.

Your first job is to convince labor that most of its members *want* workplace smoking restrictions. Show them the data gathered by the

Gallup organization and invite them to survey their own members. Convince the union that smoking is a crucial health issue and that smoking will not overshadow other workplace health concerns. In fact, because workplace smoking problems are easiest to solve and because they benefit the employer greatly in terms of increased productivity and reduced costs, workplace smoking restrictions are a stepping stone toward more safety programs. Other health and safety issues will be more easily resolved once smoking is restricted or banned. In addition, workplace smoking restrictions will create a health philosophy, a kind of mental bandwagon that carries over into other areas.

If management is initiating workplace smoking restrictions, they should notify the union of the plan and solicit comments. At every stage of the process the union should be involved and informed.

But keep in mind that no group has the moral right to prohibit workplace smoking restrictions. Unions do not have the legal right to act against limitations on smoking, because this is a health issue, not a question of privilege. Still, a union may challenge workplace smoking restrictions on the grounds that it has contractual rights to smoking areas. The Johns-Manville company won such a case against its union when a Massachusetts court ruled that the employer had both the obligation and right to protect its employees health. The National Labor Relations Board has not ruled on this issue, and it's not clear how judicial thinking will go on the subject. But, precedents and legal thought tend toward the conclusion that smoking is not subject to mandatory bargaining.

If your workplace is a hospital, these techniques can be supplemented by reports directed to meetings of medical and surgical departments and presentations to the hospital's executive committee. In addition, you can poll patients.

Sample Corporate Policies

Different companies, obviously, have developed different workplace smoking policies. Below are some examples of what various companies have approved:

Campbell Soup Company has long prohibited smoking at the workplace during normal working hours. Employees may smoke outdoors or in designated areas in the cafeteria or in plant "break" areas. Employees are informed of this 120-year-old policy during their orientation session.

City Federal prohibits smoking in all work areas except completely enclosed private offices. During meetings in these offices, the rights of nonsmokers are to be upheld. Areas prohibited include all common spaces, meeting rooms, rest rooms, hallways, stairways, and elevators.

City permits smoking in cafeterias and lounges, as long as there are no-smoking sections. The company continually monitors the quality of air throughout its facilities. In buildings that don't have lounges or cafeterias, management designates sections of the workplace where smoking is permitted, but "in every case common courtesy should guide employees who wish to take advantage of areas where smoking is allowed."[29]

Goodyear Aerospace's workplace smoking restrictions went into effect in 1986. Smoking is allowed at work stations and open building areas, except where specifically prohibited for "product specifications, processes, safety, or fire hazards."[30] In cafeterias and lunchrooms, smoking is allowed only in smoking sections. Smoking is not allowed in rest rooms at any time, and is discouraged in conference and meeting rooms. Employees who are affected by tobacco smoke report their problems to the appropriate district manager, and *"If a satisfactory accommodation cannot be made, preferences of the nonsmoking employees will prevail and smoking will be prohibited in that work area."* (Emphasis added.)

IBM has strict workplace smoking restrictions. At IBM, smoking is not allowed in confined areas including copier rooms, elevators, small terminal rooms, stairwells, shuttle buses, medical waiting and examination rooms, all waiting lines, and food-service areas. Smoking is also not permitted at meetings and classes (except when senior management decides that these rooms have adequate ventilation as determined by IBM's Real Estate and Construction Division). In addition, in common work areas and in offices that are occupied by two or more people, "the manager will make reasonable accommodations if one of the occupants objects to smoking. *If this cannot be done, smoking will be banned in these offices."* (Emphasis added.)

When *New England Bell* decided to ban smoking they implemented their policy in phases. Stage one banned smoking in conference rooms, classrooms, and company vehicles with two or more occupants. At that time arrangements were made for smokers and nonsmokers in cafeterias and lounges. Stage two, which began six months later, prohibited smoking in all work areas, including private offices. New England Telephone also sponsors programs to help smokers who want to quit.

USG Acoustical Products has forbidden its employees to smoke at work or at home. The policy was instituted for health reasons because corporate managers realized that nonsmokers have fewer sick days than smokers. The firm is also offering quit-smoking programs.[31]

Hundreds of other businesses also do not allow smoking at any work stations. Period. For many organizations this is the simplest and most intelligent solution. It's easy to enforce and understand; no smoking at work is unambiguous. Some of the firms that have instituted this policy include: *Aetna Life and Casualty, AT&T, Brooklyn District Attorney's Office* (New York), *CIGNA Insurance, Control Data Corporation, Grumman Corporation, Harvard University, Honeywell, Inc., Perkin-Elmer Corporation, Pratt & Whitney Aircraft*, and *The Wall Street Journal*.

Pacific Bell does not allow smoking anywhere at all. Neither does *The Aerobics Center* (Dallas, Texas), *the American Heart Association, the American Lung Association, all schools in Andover, Kansas, and Benton, Arkansas, the Boyde Coffee Company, British Columbia Hydro and Power Authority, Billy Graham Associates, the Holden, Massachusetts, Police Department, Kansas Gas and Electric, Johns-Manville* (Denver and New Jersey), *Logo Computer, Lyle Stuart, Inc., Minnesota Vikings football club, Newport Daily News, Northwestern Bell Telephone Company, WRNJ* in Hackettstown, New Jersey, *Zycad, Inc.*, and hundreds of other companies.

Union Mutual Life Insurance Company puts its policy on smoking this way: "Very simply stated: Effective January 1, 1986, smoking will not be permitted in company facilities, home office or field." Union Mutual offers comprehensive quit-smoking programs for its smoking employees who want to stop.

The Alexandria, Virginia, Fire Department does not hire smokers. Neither do *the Arlington and Fairfax County* (Virginia) *Fire and Police Departments, John Eastman Property Designs, Fortunoff, Johns-Manville, Northern Life Insurance Company, Radar Electric, the Salem, Oregon, Fire Department, Vanguard Electronic Tool Company* (Seattle, Washington), and hundreds of other small and large organizations.

Implementing a Nonsmokers' Rights Policy

Implementation is crucial. A poorly enforced or inconsistent policy on smoking will create numerous problems and even raise some calls for eliminating workplace smoking restrictions and going back to the dark ages of darkening lungs. And you can be sure that the Tobacco Institute will focus on even the minutest problem you may have with your nonsmoking policy, especially if yours is a large organization. The Tobacco Institute *needs* companies to encourage workplace smoking restrictions to fail, in order for them to claim that the best policy is no policy at all.

From the moment you decide to institute workplace smoking restrictions you must campaign to educate people about 1) smoking and health and 2) the elements of the policy. This information should be posted on company bulletin boards and distributed to all employees. It's worthwhile printing a brochure about smoking and health, which includes questions and answers about smoking, and tells employees why the policy has *changed* since they started work here. Be sure to focus on tobacco smoke—the culprit—not the tobacco smoker. Every memo about smoking should be signed by a corporate officer or by local management; people respond better when they know who is making the rules. Smokers and nonsmokers have to be continually informed about the policy; education should persist through the life of the program. It's a good idea to let employees know how the firm's productivity is improving because of this policy and it's an even better idea to let all employees share monetarily in the increased productivity.

No-smoking areas need to be clearly marked. *No Smoking* signs should be posted at the entrance to all areas where smoking is not allowed and inside these areas. Signs should be especially conspicuous to visitors. *No Smoking* signs don't have to be drab, by the way; they can be in any of several colors and can have illustrations on them. There's nothing to prevent you from designing a creative, attractive *No Smoking* sign—in fact, you should.

Whether the policy is implemented in phases or all at once, stick to the dates you've selected. Post a reminder the day before and the day that the limitations take effect.

Include as many supportive measures as possible. Face-to-face talks between smokers and company officers are an especially good idea. Workshops and video presentations are also helpful. Local nonsmokers' rights organizations and the heart, lung, and cancer associations can provide some of this information.

Continually monitor your program. If smokers are having trouble not smoking, talk with them. Explain the importance of everyone adhering to the restrictions and let them know that they will be enforced. Discuss how this benefits the organization; point out quit-smoking programs. If employees are clamoring for more restrictions, don't let them down. Eventually, you may discover, that the best policy for your organization is no smoking anywhere.

What happened at the Provident Indemnity Life Insurance Company is a good illustration of the path a company can take when its management supports nonsmokers' rights. Provident changed from a company that allowed smokers and nonsmokers to work together to a firm that requires employees to agree that if they smoke at all they will pay an additional $300 a year for insurance coverage. In 1980, Provident's actuarial tables listed nonsmokers as having longer life expectancies and healthier lives than smokers, and the company offered discounts as high as 33 percent on premiums for nonsmokers. When John Reese became Provident's president in 1982, he appointed a committee comprised mostly of smokers to make recommendations on how the company should manage smoking. Reese told the committee that the company's eventual goal was to become smokefree. After studying and deliberating, the committee recommended initially making all work stations, including offices, smokefree, and confining smoking to the cafeteria. For an hour a day the cafeteria would be turned into a no-smoking area. The committee also discovered that only 35 percent of Provident's 120 employees were smokers. They recommended a complete ban on smoking by the fall of 1983. The policy also included letting prospective employees know about Provident's smoking rules and offering smoking-cessation programs for employees and their spouses on company time. In September 1983 Provident barred smoking entirely on its premises and instituted its program of requiring off-the-job smokers to pay additional insurance to cover their greater health costs.

Absenteeism dropped sharply after the policy was implemented; almost no complaints have been received about it. John Reese estimated that Provident saved between $15,000 and $20,000 in cleaning and damage costs in the first year after the ban. Reese said, "Although some people were initially upset with the ban, almost everyone seems pleased with the results. Some of the pregnant women who quit smoking are particularly happy that the company adopted a policy that got them to quit smoking.'' Provident now offers a comprehensive wellness program.

MSI Insurance, of Arden Hills, Minnesota, followed a similar path. In 1983, the company embarked on a policy that eventually led to a total ban on smoking fourteen months later (save for one area of the cafeteria). Statistics on smoking helped convince smokers in management and elsewhere that this was the best course for MSI. They offered a vigorous smoking-cessation program to precede and accompany their smoking restrictions. The program began on November 17, 1983, with MSI Cold Turkey Day, during which smokers were encouraged not to smoke for twenty-four hours—or longer. Employees who didn't smoke for the day were eligible for a drawing for a frozen turkey; nonsmokers were also eligible if they signed up a smoker. As adherents to the philosophy that nonsmoking policies don't have to be harsh or bureaucratic, but can be fun, MSI handed out survival kits containing candy cigarettes, sugarless gum, and lemon drops for Cold Turkey Day. On November 17, MSI removed all its cigarette vending machines. In December, more turkeys were awarded to new nonsmokers and their sponsors, and in May smokers who had stayed off the weed for six months were eligible for a drawing for membership in a YMCA. MSI awarded $60, half the cost of the firm's smoking cessation program, to employees who successfully completed the seven-week course. Employees who quit smoking for a year were entered in a drawing for a weekend vacation—additional prizes were given out during the year.

One of the world's largest employers, the government of the United States, unveiled its policy toward smoking in the workplace in December 1986. Starting February 8, 1987, agency heads had to provide a ''reasonable smokefree environment'' for workers. This policy, which effects about a million employees and 6,900 buildings, requires local heads of agencies to separate smokers from nonsmokers and to post signs where smoking is permitted. The GSA said that generally, open workplaces must be no-smoking areas, offices can be designated smoking only if the office can be ''configurated so as to limit the involuntary exposure of nonsmokers to secondhand smoke to a minimum.'' The only offices in which smoking is permitted are offices ''large enough and sufficiently ventilated to provide separate smoking and nonsmoking sections which protect the nonsmokers against involuntary exposure to smoke,'' the regulations declare. Areas in which smoking is generally not allowed include auditoriums, classrooms, conference rooms, elevators, lobbies, rest rooms, clinics, corridors, and libraries. Cafeterias must have separate no-smoking areas. According to Constance J. Horner, director of the Office of Personnel Management, the employer is expected to save a considerable amount of money in reduced insurance costs and absenteeism. Horner added, "the employer in this case is the U.S. taxpayer."

The pro-nonsmokers' rights movement has a long tradition in American labor. Thomas Edison himself refused to hire smokers. And look at what he accomplished!

NOTES

(1) *A Decision Maker's Guide to Reducing Smoking at the Worksite*, U.S. Department of Health and Human Services, Office on Smoking and Public Health, 1985. Original source: U.S. Department of Health, Education, and Welfare, 1979.
(2) National Center for Health Statistics, 1979.
(3) *Personnel*, May 1986.
(4) *Newsday*, April 4, 1988, p. B7.
(5) James Replace, testimony before the U.S. Senate, Subcommittee on Civil Service, Post Office, and General Services, Committee on Governmental Affairs, September 30, 1985.
(6) *The Health Consequences of Smoking: Cancer and Chronic Lung Disease in the Workplace*, Surgeon General's report, 1985.
(7) J. Replace, D. Seba, A. Lowrey, and T. Gregory, "Effect of Negative Ion Generators on Ambient Tobacco Smoke," *Clinical Ecology*, Winter 1983/84, pp. 91–92.
(8) Marvin M. Kristein, "How Much Can Business Expect to Profit from Smoking Cessation?" *Preventive Medicine*, December 1983, p. 368.
(9) *It Can Be Done!: A Smokefree Workplace*, Group Health Cooperative of Puget Sound, 1985.

(10) Health Interview Survey, National Center for Health Statistics, 1974.

(11) *The Washington Post,* September 22, 1986, p. A8.

(12) James Schultz, "Perspectives on the Economic Magnitude of Cigarette Smoking," *New York State Journal of Medicine,* July 1985, p. 304.

(13) David Smith, "Absenteeism and Presenteeism in Industry," *Archives of Environmental Health,* November 1970.

(14) *Congressional Quarterly,* January 21, 1977.

(15) *Richmond Times Dispatch,* April 27, 1986, p. H1.

(16) *The Wall Street Journal,* March 17, 1987, p. 1.

(17) Martin Dewey, *Smoke in the Workplace,* Non-Smokers' Rights Association, Toronto, Canada, 1985, Dow Chemical internal report cited.

(18) Regina W. Herzlinger, "How Companies Tackle Health Care Costs: Part III," *Harvard Business Review,* January/February 1986, p. 70.

(19) Jeff Day, staff editor of the Bureau of National Affairs, testimony before the Subcommittee on Health and the Environment, Committee on Energy and Commerce, June 27, 1986.

(20) *The New York Times,* February 22, 1987, p. C12.

(21) 66 Labor Arb. Rep. 498 January 28, 1976.

(22) *Shimp v. New Jersey Bell Telephone Company,* 368 A.2d 408.

(23) 690 F.2d 731, 9th Circuit Court of Appeals, October 21, 1982.

(24) 7667-5-11, December 8, 1986.

(25) *Batchelor v. Fresno County, California,* 1982.

(26) W.D. Wash. No. C81-85

(27) *Harriett Brooks v. Transworld Air Lines and Liberty Mutual Ins. Company,* 76 SF 257-975.

(28) *The Washington Post,* November 11, 1985, p. A1.

(29) Alfred J. Hedden, City Federal president and CEO, memorandum, April 22, 1985.

(30) Goodyear memo, July 26, 1985.

(31) *The New York Times,* January 21, 1987, p. A16.

CHAPTER 7

Defending Yourself Against Tobacco Smoke

You have just finished one of the finest meals of your life at one of the best restaurants in town. You're kind of sitting back and you've got a fresh cup of coffee that's just been delivered and you light this [cigar] up. The next thing you know, there's a tap, tap, tap, tap, tap on your shoulder. You turn around and there's this person that says, "Would you mind terribly not smoking?" Your response would be?

Hold your breath until I'm done.

Dialog between Ken Schramm and
Ed Larson, representative for
the State Retail Tobacco
Dealers' Association, KOMO-TV, Seattle,
October 26, 1986

It's going to be a while before every city, town, and state has its own nonsmokers' rights laws—or before there's federal legislation protecting nonsmokers. When a smokefree society does happen, nonsmokers will no longer have to be in the awkward position of asking smokers not to light up. Nonsmokers will no longer be worried that the person they're tapping on the shoulder might hurl insults or a fist their way. Nonsmokers won't encounter people like Ed Larson of the Tobacco Dealers' Association who tells smokers to "Hold your breath until I'm done." So in the interim, we're all going to have to rely on personal strategies for clearing the air around us. Although each individual smoker and each situation will be a little different, there are some standard defensive techniques that can help you breathe clean air.

Because it's no simple feat to ask a stranger not to smoke, and because smokers are not always polite or courteous about their habit, you should develop a staple of techniques for asking smokers to refrain.

In order to breathe clean air you must always assert yourself—assert your rights. Breathing healthful air is a right. You shouldn't feel that your request that somebody put out his cigarette is a rude intrusion, an extraordinary demand, a violation of privacy, uniquely offensive, a hardship or anything like that. No. Just the opposite is true. It's the smoker's cigarette fumes that are the annoying *and dangerous* intrusion. That person, though without thinking—and that's the problem—is doing something wrong and harmful. How wrong is it? Exposing nonsmokers, especially children, pregnant women, former smokers, people with allergies, asthma, and other lung diseases, to cigarette smoke is so wrong that it is becoming illegal in many states and localities. It's very wrong. Surgeon General C. Everett Koop put it this way:

> We now have evidence that is pretty solid. In fact, the evidence is more solid in this report [the 1986 report on the health consequences of passive smoking] than it was for Luther Terry's report. Now instead of people saying, "You know, smoking annoys me, it irritates me, my sinuses ache at night and my eyes burn and my clothes smell," they can also say, "We now have solid evidence that this is dangerous to my health."

Jessica Griffith, a graphic artist at the American Pharmacological Association, is a nonsmoker. All she wants is to be able to breathe clean air. Her experiences are those of a typical nonsmoker:

> I used to feel this is an outrage and these people are slowly killing me against my will. In the last couple of years I've developed a sneezing response, an allergy; when people smoke around me it doesn't take longer than five minutes before I start sneezing. People didn't take me seriously before.
>
> I know for certain that smoking makes me sneeze. I've gone as far as tipping the maître d' ten bucks to move a cigar smoker

to another section. In the past I used to turn to people and ask them to put cigarettes out; I've even gone to get security on the Metro. Once I went to Denny's for breakfast in the no-smoking section, and there was someone smoking in the no-smoking section. So I had to ask the manager to ask that person to put his cigarette out. It worked for a few minutes, but then he lit up again. I actively avoid going to places where there is going to be cigarette smoke, such as bars.

I don't think no-smoking sections are the answer in restaurants, because the smoke drifts around.

There's enough information around to make people wonder: Why do we let people smoke around other people?

Columnist Ellen Goodman writes, ''Sharing your air rights is a bit like giving someone permission to step on your feet or burn poison ivy incense. The smoker is the aggressor. The nonsmoker is the defender.'' So we have to learn defensive strategies.

Because most smokers aren't consciously aware that they're violating your lungs—or don't want to be aware—you have to remind them. A tiny minority of smokers will inquire ''Do you mind if I smoke?'' (that's common courtesy) but most smokers think it's okay to smoke as long as nobody tells them otherwise. But it's not okay, and you should say so. Always keep this thought in mind when you wonder whether it's appropriate to ask a smoker to put his cigarette out: Cigarette smoke is damaging your lungs, making your eyes water, putting toxins in your bloodstream, irritating your throat, and turning your clothing into tobacco-soaked cloth.

In certain circumstances, you will have not only moral, but legal force behind you when you ask someone not to smoke. On a USAir flight from Buffalo, New York, to Boston in November 1986 five young men refused a pilot's order not to smoke in the no-smoking section of the plane. They were arrested by the Massachusetts state police when the plane landed. Each was fined $115 after the crew testified against them.[1]

Most smokers will put their cigarettes out promptly. Most smokers are as shy and friendly as nonsmokers and will stop once they realize that their smoke is causing problems.

It only takes a couple of seconds to ask someone not to smoke, but the benefits can last hours. You'll be happier and healthier: The few words, "Excuse me, I'd really appreciate it if you wouldn't smoke" help give your lungs a long life. As an added benefit, you may have taught that smoker to ask the people around him first before lighting up.

Restaurants

The most common setting in which common courtesy breaks down is in restaurants. Because smokers and nonsmokers alike eat out for pleasure, you should be as tactful and pleasant as possible when asking a smoker to butt out. Don't be indirect by mentioning to your dining partner in a louder than normal voice that there's smoke in the air or that smoking is unhealthy. Smokers will usually continue to puff away until you ask them not to, and when you finally broach the issue, your overheard conversation may have made them angry and defensive. Also avoid strategies like the technique one woman employed of putting her finger in a smoker's glass of water. When the astonished smoker could coax his vocal cords into asking "What was that about?" the woman responded, "If you can pollute my air, I can pollute your water." You may feel like doing that, but the approach suggested by Patrick Reynolds, grandson of the founder of R.J. Reynolds (a smoker who died of lung cancer), is much better: "I think what you have to do is smile, put a big smile on, and be very warm and say, 'That's such a nice jacket you have on. Gosh, I'd sure appreciate it if you'd put out your cigarette'—with a smile. That way, it's not so scary to tell somebody to not do something. If you can smile and ask people to stop smoking and give them an honest compliment, whatever it might be, as long as it's honest, that will help."[2]

Reynolds's suggestion, or its abbreviated variant, a pleasant, but concerned smile accompanied by a one-sentence request, "Would you mind not smoking?" is the best technique. And it's applicable to most situations.

Surgeon General Koop makes the following recommendation:

> Get involved. For too long, most nonsmokers have suffered in silence. It's time to speak up. Politely point out No Smoking signs to smokers who apparently can't read. Ask to be seated

away from smokers in restaurants. Push for local and state laws that restrict or ban smoking in public places.

Sometimes, however, you get this feeling about the smokers around you: They might not respond so responsibly to your request. Or sometimes it's essential that you avoid tobacco smoke: You have the flu, have babies with you, or have lung problems or allergies. People who are acutely affected by tobacco smoke must, in the immortal words of Star Trek's Captain James T. Kirk to his navigator, Mr. Sulu, "take evasive action." In these situations, somewhat more purposeful requests are necessary. The words you choose must convince smokers that they have to put out their cigarettes right away.

Dana Miller, a law student who is especially sensitive to tobacco smoke, developed an effective technique, which grew out of her severe allergy to tobacco. Miller must avoid tobacco smoke, and can't take the chance that a smoker will say no. She's discovered that smokers react quickly when Miller tells them that she has asthma and the tobacco fumes are going to cause an attack. No smoker wants to be responsible for directly causing illness in anyone, and they promptly put out their cigarettes. Miller also adds that she'll be finished with her meal soon.

If you are recovering from the flu or are pregnant, tell the smoker. Express the fragility of your health and thank the smoker in advance.

It's best to ask the people sitting at the tables adjacent to yours before you sit down whether they'll be smoking. This way you can create a clean air "safe zone" around your table.

Occasionally, though, it happens like this. You arrive at a restaurant where there isn't a no-smoking area. So you ask to be seated away from smokers. You tell the maître d' it's important; maybe even slip him a five-dollar bill. After surveying the restaurant for a moment, he locates a table that's isolated from smokers. In a short while, you're relaxed, and enjoying a good meal and wine when a group of four is seated at the table next to you. You hardly notice them, and you hardly notice the couple who've also just taken their chairs at the table on the other side of you. Suddenly your Bordeaux begins to taste stale, as if it's been aging in rotting wood. You put the wine down, and take a bite of your steak, which you can no longer smell. At that instant, your wife begins to cough and whispers, "The cigarette smoke is burning my eyes." Around you at two separate tables are three people puffing away on their Marlboros and Winstons. If it were just one person you might ask him not to smoke. But three? What do you do? *Ask*— definitely. You have every right to politely ask these people, a table at a time, not to smoke. It will take a minute but you should be as successful in motivating all of these people not to smoke as you would with just one individual. As always, be kind, and through your voice, gestures and eyes, let the smokers know that you understand that smoking is pleasurable. Let them know that the request is only for a short time, till you leave. Never say that their smoking is disturbing your meal, because even though it is, focusing on the annoyance aspects of tobacco smoke creates a your-pleasure-versus-their-pleasure conflict. Alternatively, ask the smokers if they could position their ashtrays to the side of the table farthest away from you. When you make this request, mention that smoking causes problems for you. Many smokers, realizing that their smoke is bothering someone, will take the initiative and put their cigarette out.

Unfortunately, more than a handful of smokers may think, "Well, my Salem may be detracting from *your* meal, but it's certainly enhancing *mine*." If you offer an explanation, mention health. It's legitimate and honest. Most smokers have a vague understanding about the link between involuntary smoking and lung disease and other disorders; for better or worse, you are part of the process of educating smokers about passive smoking. Whatever you do, *do something about tobacco smoke*. Each time you act to clear the air, you make it easier for the next nonsmoker by sensitizing smokers to the issue of sidestream smoke. In a way, you are training smokers to be considerate of nonsmokers.

Occasionally, you can achieve success through this tactic: Tell the host that you want to be seated away from smokers. Ask that the host only seat nonsmokers at the tables adjacent to yours. This is almost certainly not the first time that the maître d' has been asked to do this, but he will often have no problem seating only nonsmokers around you. In fact, it wouldn't take long to create an ad hoc no-smoking section. Fran Sauder, owner of a popular Lancaster County, Pennsylvania restaurant is typical of restaurant owners in saying, "We had so many customers who were asking for it." Ms. Sauder has turned her entire 225-seat restaurant into a no-smoking restaurant.[3] The restaurant may discover that they should have a permanent no-smoking section, after all.

If you find yourself surrounded by cigarette smoke and there's nowhere you can go, ask for a check and leave. Never suffer tobacco's effects—it's unpleasant and unhealthy. (Be sure to pay only for that which you have eaten, not everything you've ordered.) After all, you requested a table away from smokers, were escorted to that table, and now the restaurant has taken it away from you. Restaurants are service establishments, they're supposed to please you; not the other way around. If you're still reluctant to leave a restaurant that can't provide smokefree dining, think of it this way: Should you *pay money* to inhale cigarette smoke? Restaurant owners may not know about all the health effects of passive smoking, but they're certainly aware that tobacco smoke turns good food into culinary sawdust.

But there are times when you just don't feel like playing praetorian guard against smoke fumes. It is tiring, not only to ask people continually not to smoke, but to have to mentally prepare for asking. You begin to look over your shoulder furtively, you recognize certain finger movements that precede withdrawing a cigarette from a pack. It causes anxiety.

Fortunately, there are other techniques you can employ to baffle tobacco smoke.

Ahron Leichtman's approach worked successfully in Cincinnati. Leichtman, president of Cincinnati GASP and Citizens Against Tobacco Smoke, found that few restaurants offered no-smoking sections. Instead of suffering a smoky meal each time he ate out, Leichtman complained to his local newspapers. Much to his delight, Leichtman discovered that there were *many* other nonsmokers who suffered the same injustices while eating out. As a result Cincinnati GASP was formed.

The District of Columbia Lung Association manufactures adhesive stickers, measuring about a half inch by an inch that say, "I enjoyed dining here, but wish you had a NONSMOKING SECTION!"

Some nonsmokers carry small fliers that explain that passive smoking is harmful and give them to restaurant proprietors. The fliers begin, "Your cigarette smoke may be harming me . . ." and go on to talk about the effects of passive smoking on certain groups including pregnant women, the elderly, and children; they conclude with an overthanks for not smoking. Get in touch with your local Group Against Smoking Pollution, Lung, Cancer, or Heart Association about preparing an arsenal of pamphlets.

Airplanes

Things are not so murky on airplanes as they are with restaurants. Rules governing smoking on planes are very precise, and your rights are well defined. First, no flight shorter than two hours in duration may have any smoking, through 1990. (This law may be extended by Congress.) A flight is considered to be the time between take-off and landing. On flights longer than two hours in duration and on all international flights originating in the United States, you have the right to a seat in the no-smoking section of any flight, including charters, unless seats are assigned in advance *and* you are late checking in *and* there are no seats left in the no-smoking section. The airline must expand the size of the no-smoking section to meet the demands of nonsmokers. On small planes no smoking is allowed at all. If the airline doesn't offer you a no-smoking seat, it will face fines of up to $1,000 for each complaint. The basic rule is short, sweet, and reads:

(a) Except as provided by paragraph (b) of this section, air carriers, when operating aircraft designed to have a passenger capacity of 30 seats or more, shall provide as a minimum:
(1) A no-smoking area for each class of service and for charter service;
(2) A sufficient number of seats in the no-smoking sections of the aircraft for all persons who wish to be seated there;
(3) Expansion of the no-smoking sections to meet passenger demand; and
(4) Special provisions to ensure that if a no-smoking section is placed between smoking sections, the nonsmoking passengers are not unreasonably burdened.

(b) On flights for which passengers may make confirmed reservations and on which seats are assigned before boarding, an air carrier need not provide a seat in a no-smoking section to a passenger who has not met the carrier's requirement as to time and method of obtaining a seat on the flight, or who does not have a confirmed reservation. If a seat is available in the established no-smoking section, however, a carrier shall seat there any enplaning passenger who so requests, regardless of boarding time or reservation status.[4]

Speak promptly and directly when you are denied a seat in the no-smoking section. Airline personnel aren't always familiar with all the regulations affecting air travel, or if they are, they assume that passengers are not. Once you declare your rights, no employee of an airline company wants to be responsible for the company incurring a $1000 fine.

Of course the demarcation between the smoking and no-smoking sections of an airplane are far from perfect. As Dick Cavett said, "Anyone with half a brain knows that to refer to the no-smoking section of a plane is like saying the no-chlorine section of the pool." The Surgeon General describes smoke pollution on airplanes this way: "It's my suspicion that a young lady who works in the smoking end of a plane in the galley is probably 'smoking' three or four cigarettes a flight. . . . If you look back on a long flight—after dinner, especially—there is a tremendous cloud of smoke in the back, and it also is coming up to all the nonsmokers." The National Academy of Sciences, in its 1986 report *The Airliner Cabin Environment: Air Quality and Safety,* concluded that ventilation on aircraft is not sufficient to keep tobacco's gasses and particulates from drifting into the no-smoking section. In other words, people in the no-smoking section of a plane do breathe cigarette smoke. And in the Academy's words:

> Smoke exposure can become significant in aircraft with outside-airflow rates as low as 7 cfm/passenger. Even a ventilation (airflow) rate of 14–15 cfm/passenger consists of as much as 50 percent recirculated, and possibly, smoky, cabin air.

Jet aircraft keep the flow of fresh air into the aircraft to a minimum, for every cubic foot of new air circulated, more fuel is consumed. Only ventilation rates resembling gale force winds would be sufficient to clean the atmosphere in aircraft. The problem is so pervasive that the Academy recommended "a ban on smoking on all domestic flights."

The closer you are to the smoking section, the worse it gets. All this information doesn't do you much good by itself, however.

And once you're seated in the no-smoking section, you're more or less stuck there, subject to the whims of smokers behind you and vagaries of the craft's ventilation system. So planning should be two-fold. When you make your reservation, ask for a seat as far away from the smoking section as possible. A handful of airlines allow you to reserve specific seats when you make your reservation. When your tickets arrive, inspect them carefully to make sure that you're sitting in a seat in the single digits or low teens. If the airline does not have the ability or policy of reserving seats in advance, insist on it anyway. Deregulation has done many things to the airline business, but more than anything else, it's increased competition for passengers. Because the reservation clerk may not be able to accomplish this for you, you may have to contact higher authorities within the company. Don't accept a smug, "Just arrive early to get the seat you want" answer, because you don't have to. You'll probably be fumbled back and forth among supervisors, managers, perhaps even a company vice-president, until your request is satisfied. And it will be satisfied; there are no technical, legal, or real policy barriers to making special arrangements with passengers. If you're embarking on a flight midway through the plane's journey, the airline may try to tell you that they can't know which seats will be available until the plane actually takes off. True enough; then tell them that whoever assigns seats for your departure point should be given a note saying that the farthest-away seat that's available should go to you. That note should be at the check-in desk the moment the jet takes off.

Unfortunately, probably nothing you say will prevent smokers from lighting up onboard. From their perspective, the smoking section gives them unlimited rights. (Just be grateful that you're not on a European aircraft in which the smoking section is the entire left hand side of the plane!)

The second prong of attack is to write the airline after your flight and let them know that you hope they'll offer a larger no-smoking section next time, or make it easier to reserve a better no-smoking seat in advance. And while your pen is in hand, ask the airline why they don't have a no-smoking section in their waiting area, too. Airlines actually prefer that their entire craft be smokefree, because cigarette smoke increases maintenance costs and the risk of fire. Indeed, a few companies have done something about this philosophy, too. Continental Airlines initiated a trial program of giving nonsmokers a 10 percent discount on their next flight, and Air Canada has banned smoking entirely on some short flights. And small aircraft, those seating thirty or fewer passengers, manage to take off, fly, and land without smokers tearing their seats apart in a nicotine withdrawal fit.

There's one other solution: Northwest Airlines has banned smoking on all its domestic flights. Fly Northwest.

Persistence pays off. What's true for airplanes is true for airline waiting rooms. Steve Allen was spending a bit of time waiting to board a plane at San Francisco Airport. When he asked the Pan Am attendant if there was a no-smoking section in the waiting area, he smiled and pointed directly behind Allen. "Yes, Mr. Allen, there is," he said. "We've just opened one up, and I suppose you know who's partly responsible for that."

"I'm sorry," Allen said, "I have no idea who's responsible for it."

"You are," he replied. "In fact management sent around a copy of a letter that you had written, a few months ago, suggesting that we set aside some portions of the waiting room as a no-smoking area."

A letter of suggestion or complaint addressed to a corporation, worded in a civilized tone, can have an impact. And the more letters the better!

Taxis

Never feel obligated to take a taxi driven by a smoking driver. And if the driver starts smoking after you've entered the cab, politely ask him to stop. If he refuses, insist: Say you'll complain to the Taxi Commission—while they may not rule in your favor, the driver will have to spend an afternoon not working. Or, if you prefer not to be so bold, tell the driver calmly that it's okay if he wants to smoke, but then you won't feel obligated to tip him; on the other hand, you'd be grateful if he puts the cigarette out. That's fair and honest; no driver who continues to smoke in spite of his customer's pleas should be tipped. Most smoking taxi drivers would prefer to forgo a cigarette rather than a tip. Discuss this with the driver *after* you're inside the cab.

You might consider printing pamphlets about involuntary smoking and health to give to restaurant managers, cab drivers, smokers sharing the same waiting room as you, and other people who need to be educated about smoking. Give these fliers along with a "thank you" to smokers who are courteous and put their cigarettes out, and to smokers who aren't. The pamphlet should describe the Surgeon General's and National Academy of Sciences' conclusions about the dangers of passive smoking. It should also mention that nonsmokers have nothing against smoking in private, and in fact that's all you're asking for.

Receptions, bars, lounges, and other crowded areas are especially troublesome. In many cases there won't be much you can do other than leave. Each time you leave a place because of smoking, let the owner know. It may take a while, but the message will get across. If you're invited to a party or reception, when you R.S.V.P. ask if there will be no smoking. You may receive a stunned response, or no reply at all for a handful of seconds, but that question will enlighten the host. The host may do a rapid mental calculation, concluding that most of the people at the party are nonsmokers, may mentally survey the party's aftermath—filthy ashtrays, cigarette butts here and there, curtains that smell like cigarettes, a cigarette burn on a sofa—and conclude that it would be better to have a smokefree affair. No matter where you're going, always ask whether smoking will be barred. Good ideas spread quickly.

NOTES

(1) *Los Angeles Times,* November 30, 1986, p. 4.
(2) KOMO-TV, Seattle, October 26, 1986.
(3) "Anti-smoking Bill Leaves Many Huffing, Many Puffing," *Philadelphia Inquirer,* November 27, 1988, p. 1.
(4) 14 CFR Part 252.2.

CHAPTER 8

What's Next?

His right to a smoke is the same as his right to extend his fist. He's got a right to do that, until it comes into contact with my nose. Then his rights end, and my rights begin.

Congressman James Scheuer
(D–New York)

The nonsmokers' rights movement has some powerful historical analogies. In this century, the great campaigns to eliminate the scourges smallpox and polio are similar in purpose to the effort to prevent death and disease from tobacco smoke. The endeavor to put a stop to the tobacco industry's callousness toward innocent victims of secondhand smoke resembles the struggles of the 1800s and 1900s to thwart many industries' attempts to prevent the government from instituting workplace safety regulations.

Just like these great medical and public safety campaigns of the past, nonsmokers' rights are gaining ground. Once people—average citizens like you and me—become aware of the dangers of involuntary smoking, we want the government to help keep us from secondhand smoke. We want our employers to join in this effort too, by providing a safe and comfortable place to work.

Also just like the great social crusades of the past, the nonsmokers' rights movement has heroes and villains. But as this campaign grows stronger and spreads across the country, the villains become fewer, and noticeably weaker. The voices of tens of millions of Americans are loud and clear: We want to breathe healthy air!

Eventually the pro-tobacco-smoke people will become overwhelmed and silent.

But that day is not yet here. If you've succeeded in using the strategies suggested in this book to implement nonsmokers' rights in your town or workplace, don't rest there. Lend a hand to your friends in the next county, or set up a program to assist other businesses in instituting their own workplace smoking restrictions. Obtaining non-smokers' rights takes time. Smoking wasn't banned at the Olympics until the winter games in Calgary in 1988! Nonsmokers' rights benefit everyone.

There's every reason for optimism over nonsmokers' rights. Although tobacco continues to be a financial gem for the tobacco companies, the number of smokers in the country has been declining at about 2 percent a year, while the population has been rising by about 1.7 percent overall. Dozens of cities a year enact nonsmokers' rights legislation.

One of the final frontiers in the nonsmokers' rights movement is airlines. In 1988 an experimental ban on smoking went into effect, which bars cigarette smoking on all flights of less than two hours. By all accounts (except for those of the tobacco lobby), the experiment is a success: Flight attendants love the ban, and so do pilots, aircraft maintenance crews, nonsmoking passengers, and even most smokers. This successful experiment will probably lead to a ban on smoking on all flights in the United States. Northwest Airlines' ban on smoking on all domestic flights has made it very popular among nonsmokers, less so with the tobacco industry, which has decided not to fly Northwest. In Australia, a country with a large percentage of smokers, there's already a no-smoking ban on all flights, which works to everyone's satisfaction. In New Zealand, Ansett, the country's most successful airline, bans smoking, which has helped fill their seats to capacity. The chairman of Paramount Airways, a British airline, wrote to a smoking passenger who complained about their ban on smoking: "You and your wife appear to think you have a God-given right to pollute your neighbor's atmosphere. Believe me, you have not, especially when you travel on any of my hardware worth $28 million apiece." California has a ban on smoking on all in-state flights.

The atmosphere on a jet aircraft is constantly being recycled. Very little fresh air is let in during a flight, so that the concentrations of cigarette smoke increase in direct proportion to the length of a flight. Most dangerous components of tobacco smoke can't be seen or smelled and are circulated throughout the plane. By the end of a one-hour flight, toxic levels of tobacco byproducts exist throughout the aircraft. Although the first few no-smoking seats adjacent to the smoking section receive the highest exposure, there are no safe-air seats anywhere on an aircraft. Flights that exceed an hour are even worse. A total no-smoking ban on airlines will improve the comfort and health of millions of smoking and nonsmoking passengers who choose not to sit in a smoke-filled airline cabin. It will also make a great difference in the health of the seventy thousand flight attendants who are required to work in a hazardous atmosphere. Tobacco smoke on an airline is heaviest around five to six feet high—about the head height of flight attendants. Between 5 to 10 percent of them suffer from respiratory problems caused by involuntary smoking.[1] Because airlines allow pregnant women to work on airlines through early pregnancy, their fetuses are being exposed to dangerous levels of nicotine, carbon monoxide, benzopyrene, and other chemicals in cigarette smoke.

Nonsmokers' rights has gained broad acceptability. Smoking itself is looking more and more like a deviant behavior—like a stupid thing to do. There are plenty of signs of this, but one of the best is that you'll rarely find a corporate annual report displaying an executive smoking a cigarette. It doesn't go over well with stockholders. Besides, most corporate executives have quit.

What about the pro-tobacco side? What will they do next? Well, yes, Virginia Slims, there is a "Smokers' Rights" movement, too. But the so-called smokers' rights campaign is a creation of the imagination of the cigarette companies. As *The Wall Street Journal* put it:

> In its war against smoking restrictions, the tobacco industry has spent millions trying to galvanize its customers to speak out. Huge computer data bases, sophisticated phone and mail campaigns, glossy publications—they've all been employed in hopes of creating a grass-roots smokers' rights movement.
> It hasn't worked.[2]

There are plenty of reasons why the smokers' rights campaign is as solid as a whiff of cigarette smoke. Most smokers like the civility of smoking and nonsmoking sections. Most smokers like the certainty of knowing where smoking is allowed and where it isn't. More and more smokers believe that smoking adversely affects nonsmokers. Most smokers are courteous. Many smokers would like to quit, and no-smoking rules help. "Many" smokers, says *The Wall Street Journal*, "have ambivalent feelings about cigarette makers." And most smokers like to sit in no-smoking sections, too. The executive vice-president of Northwest Airlines explained his company's decision to ban smoking on all domestic flights this way: "Well over 30 percent of our smokers are requesting no-smoking seats. In fact, a large number of them say that they will choose an airline that's nonsmoking because they want a clean-air environment."[3]

Be prepared for anything. Strange things will continue to happen in the struggle for nonsmokers' rights. In Roanoke, Virginia, a sixteen-year-old was fired from his part-time job at the Cystic Fibrosis Foundation because he couldn't tolerate his coworkers' smoking. After considerable embarrassment on the part of the local foundation, the boy was offered his job back.[4]

The future belongs to those who work to create it. The future will see lower lung cancer rates, lower heart disease rates, lower emphysema rates, and better health for all Americans. The nonsmokers' rights movement has so much momentum that it's no longer a question if smoking will be restricted in public places and office spaces, but when this will happen.

The tobacco industry is feeling the tide of this movement. As *The New York Times* wrote, "Battered by growing bans on public smoking and a recent court decision finding a tobacco company liable in the death of a smoker, the nation's largest cigarette maker is planning to spend up to $5 million in an advertising campaign that will emphasize the economic power of smokers."[5] Philip Morris's ads have appeared and amounted to nothing. They've had no effect on elections and no effect on the passage of nonsmokers' rights laws.

One final question remains to be answered: What would happen if smoking were eliminated, period? What would be the consequences of fifty million Americans kicking the habit? In terms of lives, these smokers would live an average of ten years longer. Thousands of nonsmokers would avoid disease and death from being exposed to tobacco. Absenteeism would drop at the workplace.

And what about the net effects on the U.S. economy? What about all that lost tax revenue? It would easily be made up in the amount people would save on cigarettes, some $500 a year, which could be plowed back into the economy through savings or purchases of other products.[6]

How would tobacco farmers fare? Ultimately many would have to switch from tobacco to other crops, but this change would come gradually over generations. Surprisingly, neither tobacco farmers, nor the tobacco industry would die out if cigarette consumption in the United States ended, or dropped dramatically. For while the percentage of smokers in the United States is declining (from 42.2 percent of the U.S. population in 1966 to 26.5 percent in 1986), the number of people who smoke U.S.-made cigarettes around the world is growing. In 1987 roughly 100 billion American cigarettes were exported; the figure was only 64 billion the previous year.

The tobacco industry will continue to delay its decline in a myriad of unpredictable, and often, unprofitable ways. In 1988 RJR Nabisco test-marketed a "smokeless cigarette" called Premier, a cigarette that did not produce smoke as a byproduct. Partly to try to get around the complaints of nonsmokers, and partly to alleviate some of the fear of cancer among smokers, R.J. Reynolds thought that this cleaner cigarette was a terrific idea. RJR was immediately assaulted on two fronts: The health community called this product what it was, a nicotine delivery system (actually, in its patent RJR said that the device "may be modified for use as drug delivery articles"), and petitioned the Federal Drug Administration to curtail its sale. And the marketplace didn't seem to be buying.

Will smoking on airlines continue to be a controversial issue? Perhaps a combined assault on two fronts will nip this problem in the bud: A total airline smoking prohibition will help alleviate the uncertainty about airline smoking and the opportunities for misinterpretation about regulations. But a surprise assist may come from technology: A nicotine pill popped before a flight can reduce smokers' craving for tobacco. After all, it's the nicotine in cigarettes that smokers are addicted to.

Whatever happens in the nonsmokers' rights movement, we must not become complacent. The tobacco industry won't give up. They have plenty of money, plenty of political influence and plenty of smarts. A few victories for nonsmokers' rights here and there do not make for winning the war against the cigarette companies. Nonsmokers' rights will only benefit everyone when smoking is banned in public everywhere.

It's important to remember that the nonsmokers' rights movement is not a battle between the tobacco companies and nonsmokers. It's not even a conflict between smokers and nonsmokers. The message of the nonsmokers' rights movement is not to stop the production and consumption of cigarettes in the United States. It is simply a struggle for basic human rights: the right to live a healthy life. That's worth fighting for.

NOTES

(1) "Flying America's Smoky Skies," Tony Lang, *The Cincinnati Enquirer*, July 19, 1987, p. I2.
(2) "Smokers' Rights Campaign Suffers From Lack of Dedicated Recruits," Alix M. Freedman, *The Wall Street Journal*, April 11, 1988, p. 29.
(3) A.B. Magary, *This Week with David Brinkley*, NBC-TV, March 27, 1988.
(4) *Richmond Times Dispatch*, February 13, 1988, p. B3.
(5) "New Ads by Philip Morris Stress Power of Smokers," *The New York Times*, June 29, 1988, p. 1.
(6) "On Banning Tobacco Advertising," Noel McAfee, Master's Thesis, Duke University, April 1987.

APPENDIX A

Who's Who in the Nonsmokers' Rights Movement

Action on Smoking and Health
2013 H Street, N.W.
Washington, D.C. 20006
(202) 659-4310

John F. Banzhaf, III, President
Athena Mueller, Legal Counsel

Action on Smoking and Health is the oldest organization in America that focuses exclusively on tobacco smoking. ASH was founded by its current president, John F. Banzhaf III, a professor of law at Georgetown University, and a man who is famous for his steadfast opposition to tobacco smoking and achievements in protecting the health of nonsmokers. If there's one group the tobacco industry fears more than any other it's ASH. When people think of a crusader against cigarette smoking, they think of John Banzhaf. His moral center is unwavering. Back in the days when television and radio advertising of cigarettes was legal, ASH was responsible for requiring television and radio stations to offer equal time to antismoking commercials, which resulted in the most dramatic decline in smoking since Surgeon General Luther Terry's original report on smoking and health in 1964. Banzhaf and the no-smoking community were awarded some $200 million in free airtime by the Federal Communications Commission. ASH broke the story on the smokeless cigarette. Children who smoke have also been a target of

ASH's efforts. ASH fought for strengthened warnings on cigarette packages and advertising. We can also thank ASH for the ban on cigar and pipe smoking on airplanes, for no-smoking sections on aircraft and for encouraging strict enforcement of nonsmokers' rights in the air.

ASH is a nonprofit, tax-exempt organization.

Banzhaf organized the first World Conference on Nonsmokers' Rights, held in Washington, D.C., in 1985. ASH publishes a newsletter, *ASH Review,* on smoking and health which contains valuable information about legal, legislative, medical, economic, and social aspects of smoking and nonsmokers' rights.

ASH's goals include seeking a ban on smoking on all planes at all times, banning smoking in the workplace and other indoor spaces, prohibiting advertising of tobacco products, and educating people about the harmful effects of smoking.

ASH offers valuable reference material to individuals and groups concerned with nonsmokers' rights. In addition to *ASH Review,* Action on Smoking and Health has material that can assist in organizing and educating people about nonsmokers' rights. Also available are buttons, stickers, and pamphlets. One of ASH's most useful publications is a pocket guide to nonsmokers' rights on airplanes: This handy card can be used to defend your rights when airline personnel say "Sorry—there are no more seats in the no-smoking section."

American Cancer Society
3340 Peachtree Road, N.E.
Atlanta, GA 30026
(404) 320-3333

The American Cancer Society is a medical and research organization. It provides comprehensive literature on the risks of passive smoking. The national office will put you in touch with local chapters if you are interested in helping the Cancer Society or if you need information about smoking and cancer. The Society works closely with the Lung and Heart associations in a three-group antismoking coalition, called the Coalition on Smoking or Health. Dr. Robert V.P. Hunter, M.D., of the Cancer Society, says, "Exposure to involuntary smoke increases the risk of lung cancer about 30 percent. Among those heavily exposed, the risk increases 100 percent.'' The American Cancer Society also provides information on all types of cancers and their treatment, and sponsors a National Cancer Hotline.

American Heart Association
1250 Connecticut Ave., N.W.
Suite 360
Washington, D.C. 20036
(202) 822-9380

The American Heart Association has long been a champion of the antismoking movement. Its actions stem from a medical point of view: Smoking causes heart disease. More recently the Heart Association has become involved with the nonsmokers' rights movement because of the evidence that involuntary smoking causes heart disease in otherwise healthy nonsmokers. Scott Ballin, vice president of the American Heart Association, says, ''Smokers are jeopardizing the health of their families, their colleagues at work, and others by exposing them to cigarette smoke.'' Dr. Stuart F. Seides, M.D., of the Heart Association added, ''There is an increased risk of heart disease both in nonsmoking men and nonsmoking women who are married to smokers . . . The more the spouse smokes, the greater the heart disease risk to the nonsmoker.''

With the Coalition on Smoking or Health, the Heart Association is working for a Tobacco Free Young America Project.

American Lung Association
1740 Broadway
New York, NY 10019
(212) 315-8700

In 1985, the ALA was called by Jane Brody of *The New York Times,* ''a champion of nonsmokers' rights. The ALA is very active in legislation and regulation of nonsmokers rights' laws. According to Michele Kling, ''Founded in 1904, the Lung Association's original purpose was to fight tuberculosis. As tuberculosis receded as a major plague, a new plague of smoking-related lung diseases has come about, so we have turned our attention to that. Cigarette smoking has been the number one priority of the ALA since the early 1980s.''

There are over 250 local Lung Associations throughout the United States. To get in touch with the ALA, says Kling, "just look in the white pages under American Lung Association."

The ALA can provide you or your nonsmokers' rights group with information on the health hazards of smoking. If you are forming a nonsmokers rights' group, the ALA can help you in passing legislation by giving you detailed information about lobbying on local legislation. The ALA can also provide films, quit-smoking materials, and information on local ordinances.

The Lung Association works closely with the American Heart Association and the American Cancer Society. In many localities a coalition of these three groups will be actively pursuing legislation to get nonsmokers' rights. Kling says, "If you are interested in influencing federal legislation, be sure to lobby your congressmen. It's important to make your wishes for nonsmokers' rights known to your representatives and senators. Every time you read that there's going to be a vote in congress on smoking, write your representatives."

ALA has a program called "Freedom from Smoking at Work." The local Lung Association will send a consultant to your workplace to develop a workplace policy that's satisfactory to everyone. They will work with management and employees to develop a program specifically tailored to your needs. It could be anything from a total ban on smoking to a ban on smoking in certain areas. The ALA will conduct a clinic on how to quit smoking, and provide manuals and brochures. It's a "comprehensive plan" that "makes employees feel good about the process because everyone is involved." The program has grown dramatically since 1985 when the ALA conducted a Gallup poll indicating that 79 percent of all smokers and nonsmokers want workplace smoking restriction.

Americans for Nonsmokers' Rights
2054 University Avenue, Suite 500
Berkeley, CA 94704
(415) 841-3032

Walt Bilofsky, President
Mark Pertschuk, Executive Director
Julia Carol, Associate Director

Originally Californians for Nonsmokers' Rights, Americans for Nonsmokers' Rights has grown into a national organization. The organization's goal is to implement nonsmokers' rights laws throughout the country. Americans for Nonsmokers' Rights publishes a newsletter, and provides a wealth of valuable information on smoking, health, and the legislative aspects of nonsmokers' rights. ANR monitors nonsmokers' rights legislation around the country and updates what's happening in their quarterly newsletter. The group also publishes books and brochures including *Smokefree Travel Guide,* by Julia Carol; *Tobacco Smoke and the Nonsmoker; Ticket for Smokefree Flight,* which answers questions about smoking and flying; *Educate Our Kids for Life,* which talks about educating kids about smoking; *Legislative Approaches to a Smokefree Society;* curriculum guides for antismoking films; a booklet called "A Smokefree Workplace," the confidential Federal Trade Commission report on tobacco; a national listing of local smoking ordinances; and a list of the nonsmokers' rights groups around the country.

According to Julia Carol, "We are the only national nonsmokers' rights group that lobbies and that designs, creates, and implements smoking curricula. We are in business to go out of business. Our goal is to win and be done with it. As difficult as things are, we think we are going to succeed in our goal, which is to protect nonsmokers from breathing secondhand smoke."

She added, "We work closely with the nonsmokers' rights groups around the country. The nonsmokers' rights groups are great.

"This whole issue has been a grass-roots social movement. Fifteen years ago there was a Benson and Hedges ad where someone got a cigarette caught in an elevator door. Back then it was socially acceptable behavior to smoke in an elevator. In fifteen years that's changed dramatically—now there's practically no place where you can smoke in an elevator.

"We feel responsible to our members. We feel that we are here to get smoke out of their faces as soon as possible.

"We're lucky because we can respond immediately. We don't have to go through committees. We are sort of a lean, clean fighting machine.

"To get a smokefree society we have to first raise a generation of nonsmokers."

If ANR has a motto, it is this: Walker Merryman of the Tobacco Institute said that being attacked by the nonsmokers' rights movement is "like being pecked to death by ducks." Americans for Nonsmokers' Rights says, "Keep on pecking. In a fight between a duck and an elephant, bet on the elephant. In a fight between a thousand ducks and an elephant, bet on the ducks."

Basic membership is $25 a year.

Citizens Against Tobacco Smoke
P.O. Box 36236
Cincinnati, Ohio 45236
(513) 984-8833

Ahron Leichtman, President

Citizens Against Tobacco Smoke (CATS) is a relative newcomer to the nonsmokers' rights movement, although its president, Ahron Leichtman, has been involved with nonsmokers' rights since 1977. Leichtman is an independent motion picture producer and writer who coordinated the public relations campaign for Proposition Five, the California Clean Indoor Air Act of 1978. Proposition Five was the first statewide nonsmokers' rights initiative to be placed on a ballot before the electorate. "I'm not trying to keep the Marlboro man from smoking. I'm just trying to keep him on his own range," says Leichtman.

CATS is a national coalition of antismoking organizations whose goal is a smokefree society and whose approach involves coordinating antismoking legislation around the country. CATS is focusing on banning smoking on all airplanes and creating an antismoking curriculum to encourage children not to smoke. One of CATS' objectives is to unite pilots and other flight personnel against smoking—which not only is a chronic health hazard, but can cause fires in aircraft. The organization also called on former baseball commissioner Peter Ueberroth to offer no-smoking sections in baseball stadiums.

CATS can provide individuals who want to start nonsmokers' rights groups, as well as existing GASPs, with organizing, media, and lobbying support, including technical advice. Membership in CATS is $20 per year. Attractive no-smoking pins, showing a cigarette inside the universal ban symbol—a circle with a red slash through it—are available from CATS for $5.

Doctors Ought to Care (DOC)
DOC National Office
1423 Harper Street
Augusta, GA 30912

Alan Blum, M.D., founder

Doctors Ought to Care (DOC) is the oldest physicians' health promotion group in the United States, and the foremost physicians' antismoking organization. When Dr. Alan Blum started the group in 1977 with just three doctors, its purpose was to educate the public, especially youth, "in refreshing and humorous ways" about the major preventable causes of poor health and high medical costs. DOC went about purchasing advertising to counter both. DOC prefers advertising to public service announcements. According to Dr. Blum, the "problem with public service ads is that they say things like 'don't talk to strangers' at three A.M., when only the strangers are watching."

Dr. Blum said, "I started DOC as a way to tap the highest possible level of commitment of health professionals." DOC now has five thousand physician members.

DOC sticks to its themes, creating innovative, bittersweet projects. "We sponsored the US Boomerang Team after we heard that they were going to be sponsored by Philip Morris," says Dr. Blum. When Philip Morris sponsored an essay competition on the first amendment, DOC sponsored its own essay contest with a $1,000 prize for the best answer to the question, "Are tobacco company executives responsible for the deaths, diseases, and fires their products cause?" DOC is planning more essay competitions with even more compelling questions such as, "What would you like to see as the ideal punishment for a tobacco company executive?" and "What should be the best way to counteract tobacco industry tactics in developing countries?" DOC also sponsors an ongoing competition throughout the year for the best counters to cigarette advertising, called the DOC P-U competition. Dr. Blum described the competition this way: "We don't accept antismoking ads, but we counter imaging. We are looking for ways to ridicule their images. One way could be as simple as drawing a mustache on the Virginia Slims woman. Instead of Virginia Slims you get Emphysema Slims Tennis Tournament."

If you're interested in entering the DOC P-U contest send a stamped, self-addressed envelope to DOC.

Dr. Blum wants "to get people to think about tobacco in a different way." He says, "The danger is that people believe that we are doing so well against smoking—but that's not true, especially for minority and low-income groups."

For Dr. Blum and DOC the problem is the tobacco companies. "I don't use the term nonsmoker. I talk about people who smoke and people who don't. When you use the term smokers and nonsmokers you get the sense that the world is divided into smokers and nonsmokers. I don't think we should categorize the world into smokers and nonsmokers. That's what the tobacco companies want. If we let the tobacco companies divide the world like that, we lose."

The cigarette industry likes people to believe that the nonsmokers' rights movement is made up of a bunch of people who want to control the way others live. Dr. Blum has a different point of view: "The tobacco companies are the ones telling everyone what to do. The leading advertised product in America is cigarettes. If you count up the number of images a year—at ball games, point-of-purchase displays, billboards, magazines—all of those add up to far more than all the antismokers telling people what to do. But in our society we don't identify advertising as telling people what to do."

Dr. Blum likes to compare the cigarette companies to a disease. "Here is an analogy: If you study AIDS, you study the AIDS virus, the vector. If you study smoking, all you get is tips on how to quit, once you've been infected. But how do you get infected? Well, you don't pick one up on the street. That's the problem. We are so used to this problem, smoking—we think it's normal. It's not normal. It's harmful. You have a parasitic disease called the cigarette industry."

Health professionals may join DOC by contacting the national office.

Tobacco Products Liability Project
Northeastern University
School of Law
400 Huntington Avenue
Boston, MA 02115
(617) 437-2026

The Tobacco Products Liability Project is a coalition of attorneys and activists involved in litigation against the tobacco companies. The groups main thrust is to prove in court that cigarette companies are liable for the damage caused to smokers, and to win monetary damages against these companies. The TPLP holds an annual conference each year at which individuals involved in these various legal efforts exchange information and explore new strategies against cigarette companies. It views encouraging and supporting law suits against tobacco companies as a public health strategy.

The TPLP also collects data on smokers who have contracted diseases because of smoking. They are involved in the publication of a professional journal, the *Tobacco Products Litigation Reporter,* which costs $725 a year for nonmembers and $575 a year for TPLP contributors. For a donation of $35 or more you will receive a subscription to "Tobacco on Trial."

During the *Cipollone v. Liggett et al.* cigarette trial the TPLP made public previously confidential tobacco company documents. These documents proved, for the first time, what many people long suspected: The tobacco companies knew that smoking was harmful, but kept that information a secret.

The TPLP was founded in November 1984 by Northeastern University law professor Richard Daynard and Boston psychiatrist Michael Charney. It was founded as a project of the Clean Air Education Foundation. Its origins were the frustration that "many antismoking activists felt as a result of the slow pace of antismoking action," says Professor Daynard. "Almost nothing was being done in the legislative area. Tobacco companies were able to do anything they wanted to attract smokers and keep smokers."

The TPLP has five goals:

1. To make the price of cigarettes better reflect the social cost of using cigarettes. The TPLP hopes that successful law suits will force tobacco companies to raise the price of cigarettes to pay for self-insurance to cover the cost of paying settlements to families of smokers killed by cigarettes smoking. The TPLP notes that raising the price of cigarettes discourages teenagers from ever starting to smoke.

2. To produce dramatic publicity against dangers of smoking. Daynard says, "People tend to say statistics are statistics, not real people. What these cases have done is to humanize the effects of smoking—lung cancer, emphysema, peripheral vascular disease." Our law suits, he continued, "dramatize that these are effects that happen to real people. There is now discussion in the public about

whether the tobacco companies should be blamed for deaths—this has been very effective antismoking publicity.'' The TPLP's suits have put the cigarette industry in an embarrassing position, according to Daynard. ''What we have done is force the tobacco companies to take the position that you really have to be reckless to use their products.''

3. To initiate a Watergate-like search into what the tobacco companies know, when they knew it, and what they did about it. The Cipollone case documents were very important in this regard.

4. To provide some compensation to the families of tobacco smoking. Daynard says, ''I'm not saying that the smokers aren't partially responsible, but the companies are more responsible.'' The TPLP also hopes to pave the way for third parties to recover from cigarette companies. Third-party insurance payers can file a suit to recover money from the tobacco companies under the legal doctrine of ''subrogation clauses'' when smokers die from tobacco-inspired diseases. This would, ''equalize the real costs of smoking.''

5. To require the companies to clean up their act in terms of advertising and marketing. Hopefully, the courts will clarify the preemption doctrine that currently says the tobacco companies are protected from suits because there are warnings on cigarette packs. If this clause is clarified the tobacco companies won't be able to use the warnings on their packs to say that smokers knew smoking was harmful. If the preemption clause is clarified, the cigarette companies will have to immediately stop misleading advertising—their seductive advertising. The Tobacco Institute will have to stop saying that smoking doesn't cause cancer, because that is a type of misleading advertising. It's lying and lying is not allowed in advertising. (Daynard made the analogy that what the Tobacco Institute is doing is like the asbestos companies saying that asbestos doesn't cause lung disease—if the asbestos association said that, the government would make them retract that in an instant.)

''I see the Camel ads '75 years and still smoking' as a health claim,'' Daynard says.

You can get involved with the TPLP in several ways. First, as with all the nonsmokers' rights groups, donations are welcome. If you know of a smoker who has died from cigarette smoking, let the TPLP know. They will try to set the family up with a lawyer. Lawyers who are interested in working on tobacco suits should contact the TPLP.

STATE AND LOCAL NONSMOKERS' RIGHTS GROUPS*

ALASKA

G. Miller
GASP of Juneau
PO Box 2436
Juneau, AK 99803

GASP-Fairbanks Alaska
1782 Red Fox Drive
Fairbanks, Ak 99709

ARIZONA

Helen Chlebo
Lee Fairbanks, M.D.
Arizonians Concerned About
  Smoking
PO Box 31280
Phoenix, AZ 85046
(602) 482-0994

Betty Campbell
Arizonians for Nonsmokers'
  Rights
11436 N 37th Avenue
Phoenix, AZ 85029
(602) 938-0838

Betty Campbell
Arizonians for Nonsmokers'
  Rights
PO Box 35201
Phoenix, AZ 85069
(602) 938-0838

Charles Nugent, M.D.
Nonsmokers Inc.

PO Box 12666
Tucson, AZ 85732
(602) 323-3699

ARKANSAS

Charlotte Wallace
Clayton Blackstock
Arkansans for Nonsmokers'
  Rights
PO Box 7697
Little Rock, AR 72217
(501) 378-7870

CALIFORNIA

Allan Ake
Americans for Nonsmokers'
  Rights,
San Fernando Affiliate
PO Box 89
Van Nuys, CA 91408
(818) 881-1548

Carl Siminow
Americans for Nonsmokers'
  Rights,
Westside Affiliate
PO Box 3225
Santa Monica, CA 90403
(213) 395-8069
(213) 829-4373

Mary Ann Hansen
GASP-Petaluma

* List courtesy of Americans for Nonsmokers' Rights

1123 F Street
Petaluma, CA 94952
(707) 762-3963

Geri Howard
Santa Monica GASP
PO Box 5281
Santa Monica, CA 90405
(213) 399-4937

COLORADO

Sharon Mollica
Aspen GASP
PO Box 1594
Aspen CO, 81612
(303) 925-8990

Pete Bialick
GASP of Colorado
Box 12103
Boulder, CO 80303
(303) 444-9799

FLORIDA

Rita Zemlock
GASP of Miami
PO Box 45-0952
Miami, FL 33245
(305) 868-1003

Debby Houghton
GASP of Tampa Bay
11413 Ventura Way
Tampa, FL 33637
(803) 985-8113

Orlando GASP
PO Box 7444-A
Orlando, FL 32604

Henry Olness
Right to Breathe, Inc.
PO Box 7772
Naples, FL 33941

Dean E. Woodworth
Tallahassee GASP
3612 Londerry Drive
Tallahassee, FL 32308
(904) 893-1485

GEORGIA

Sidney Ayscue
Americans for a Smoke-Free
   Society
2175 Lenox Road NE, Suite
   A-7
Atlanta, GA 30324
(404) 299-2604

D. Gordon Draves
Georgians Against Smoking
   Poll
PO Box 45098, or
PO Box 450981
Atlanta, GA 30345
(404) 296-9526

HAWAII

Hawaiian Clean Air Team
PO Box 4349

Honolulu, HI 96813
(808) 944-0884

Dave McFaull
HINO
109 Poloke Place
Honolulu, HI 96822
(808) 946-3361

INDIANA

John R. Seffrin, Ph.D.
Indiana University
HPER Building 116
Bloomington, IN 47405

KANSAS

Wilma Major
Citizens for Clean Indoor Air
PO Box 40454
Overland Park, KS 66204
(816) 274-1321

Dave Pomeroy
Kansans for Nonsmokers'
  Rights
1169 Webster
Topeka, KS 66604
(913) 354-4963

Gary Tripp
Bonnie Booker
Wicnita GASP, Inc.
PO Box 17062
Wichita, KS 67217
(316) 685-4277

LOUISIANA

Ben Fontaine
Nonsmokers' Rights Council
  of Louisiana
333 St. Charles Avenue
  #500
New Orleans, LA 70130
(504) 523-5864

MAINE

Susan C. Lawrence
GASP of Maine
47 Thomas Street
Portland, ME 04102
(207) 775-0287

MARYLAND

John O'Hara
Bowie GASP
PO Box 863
Bowie, MD 20715
(301) 262-5867

Joan Coble
Coalition of Nonsmokers
Memorial Hospital
South Washington Street
Easton, MD 21601
(301) 833-1000

Clara Gouin
GASP
PO Box 632
College Park, MD 20740

(301) 577-6427
(301) 474-0967

Lucy Douglas
Nonsmokers' Rights Group
c/o ALA of Mid-Maryland
170 Rollins Avenue
Rockville, MD 20852
(301) 881-6852

MASSACHUSETTS

American Nonsmokers' Association
32 Glenwood Avenue
Newton, MA 02159

Jerry Maldavir
GASP of Massachusetts
25 Deaconess Road
Boston, MA 02215
(617) 266-2088

MICHIGAN

Kenneth Pingel
GASP
c/o ALA of Michigan
1925 Pauline Plaza
Ann Arbor, MI 48103
(313) 995-1030

Karen Krzanowski
ALA of Michigan
403 Seymor Avenue
Lansing, MI 48933
(517) 484-4541

Karen D. Krzanowski
1621 Dobie Circle
Okemos, MI 48864

Gerald O'Grady
Jane Conrad
People Against Tobacco
Smoke (PATS)
PO Box 4394
Auburn Hills, MI 48057
(313) 852-7287

MINNESOTA

Sandra Sandell
Association for Nonsmokers' Rights (ANSR)
1421 Park Avenue
Minneapolis MN 55404
(612) 339-1902

Jeanne Weigum
Association for Nonsmokers' Rights (ANSR)
1647 Laurel
St. Paul, MN 55104
(612) 339-1902

Michael F. Maile
Minnesota Coalition for a Smokefree Society in Year 2000
2221 University Avenue SE, #400
Minneapolis, MN 55414
(612) 378-0902

MISSOURI

Center for Nonsmokers' Rights

2007 Broadway
Kansas City, MO 64108

Martin Pion
Missouri GASP
6 Manor Lane
St. Louis, MO 63135
(314) 521-0299

Paul Smith
Missouri GASP Inc.
50 White Plains Drive
Chesterfield, MO 63017

NEW JERSEY

Regina Carlson
New Jersey GASP
105 Mountain Avenue
Summit, NJ 07901
(201) 273-9368

NEW MEXICO

GASP New Mexico
2908 Aliso Drive NE
Albuquerque, NM 87110

George Coen
GASP-New Mexico
9204 Gutoerrez
Albuquerque, NM 87111
(505) 888-4694

New Mexico Nonsmokers'
Protection Projects
PO Box 657
Los Alamos, NM 87544

Charlotte Motter
Please No Smoking Club
PO Box 25972
Albuquerque, NM 87125
(505) 892-0291

NEW YORK

Rhoda Nichter
GASP New York, Long Island Division
7 Maxine Avenue
Plainview, NY 11803
(516) 938-0080

Darlene Zelenke
New Yorkers for Nonsmokers' Rights
432 Livingston Avenue
Albany, NY 12206
(518) 436-1148

Laura Breitman
Orange County Breathes
39 Mountainside Road
Warwick, NY 10990
(914) 258-4796

Chris Godek
People for a Smokefree Indoors
122 E 57th Street, Suite 4R
New York, NY 10022
(212) 832-8858 W

Carol Waterman
Right to Breathe
18 Warren Street

McKnownville, NY 12203
(518) 489-1188

NORTH CAROLINA

Doug Hodges
North Carolina GASP
105 Higbee
Durham, NC 27704
(919) 471-0988

OHIO

Butler County GASP
6068 Happy Valley Court
Fairfield, OH 45014
(513) 829-5374

Cincinnati GASP
PO Box 37731
Cincinnati, OH 45222
(513) 984-8843

Dan Zavon
Cincinnati GASP
3516 Vine Street
Cincinnati, OH 45220
(513) 222-8391
(513) 961-4277

Dayton GASP
4150 Walshwood Court
Dayton, OH 45424
(513) 222-8391

Andy Ginsburg
Ohio GASP
PO Box 14774
Cleveland, OH 44114
(216) 321-2320

Bob Weinberg
Ohio GASP,
Akron Chapter
PO Box 8338
Akron, OH 44320
(216) 864-5037

Charles Gibson
Ohio GASP,
Canton Chapter
PO Box 8434
Canton, OH 44711
(216) 494-9607
(216) 454-1105

Ohio GASP,
Cleveland Chapter
PO Box 14871
Cleveland, OH 44114
(216) 228-1615

Barbara Stanford
Ohio GASP,
Columbus Chapter
PO Box 552
Worthington, OH 43085
(614) 885-0452
(614) 888-7394

Roger Kirkpatrick
Ohio GASP,
Marietta Chapter
927 Colegate Drive
PO Box 2163
Marietta, OH 45750
(614) 374-6732
(614) 374-4844

Ed Murphy
Ohio GASP,

Miami Valley Chapter
1747 Coventry Road
Dayton, OH 45420
(513) 258-8614

Patti H. Foley
Ohio GASP,
Toledo Chapter
PO Box 14438
Toledo, OH 43614
(419) 385-7928

PENNSYLVANIA

Vincent Romito
Association for Nonsmok-
ers' Rights of Pennsylva-
nia, Inc.
PO Box 4983
Pittsburgh, PA 15206
(412) 795-4241

Patricia Pelkofer
Pennsylvania GASP
PO Box 5156
Pittsburgh, PA 15206
(412) 441-6650

SOUTH DAKOTA

Ruth Herzberg
E. Gilchrist
Citizens Against Public
Smoking (CAPS)
517 Cedar Street
Route 2, Box 46
Hitchcock, SD 57348
(605) 266-2513
(605) 266-2786

TEXAS

Association for Clean Indoor
Air
2727 Inwood Road, #106
Dallas, TX 75235
(214) 351-2228

Mrs. Earl Moore
Caring for Nonsmokers
7022 S. Jan Mar
Dallas, TX 75230
(214) 361-6192

David Ferris
Friends of Austin Nonsmokers
PO Box 180751
Austin, TX 78718
(512) 926-9600

Craig Campbell
Craig Miller
TAPS, Inc.
PO Box 27227
Houston, TX 77227
(713) 635-3200
(713) 453-5798

Charles Gibson
Texas Association of Non-
smokers
5201 South Seventh
Abilene, TX 79605

VERMONT

Stanton A. Glantz, M.D.
114 Iroquois

Essex Junction, VT 05452
(802) 879-2038

VIRGINIA

Anne Morrow Donley
Virginia GASP
PO Box 38134
Richmond, VA 23231
(804) 795-2006

WASHINGTON

Dan Herting
Fresh Air for Nonsmokers
PO Box 25
Richland, WA 99352
(509) 373-2532
(509) 943-2518

WASHINGTON

Betsy Warder
Fresh Air for Nonsmokers
    (FANS)
3323-A Windolph
Olympia, WA 98502
(206) 866-0352

Don Moore
Fresh Air for Nonsmokers
    (FANS)
PO Box 1357
Spokane, WA 99210
(509) 926-6033

Ray Paolella
Fresh Air for Nonsmokers

(FANS)
419 South 27th Avenue
Yakima, WA 98902
(509) 248-4005

Robert Fox
Fresh Air for Nonsmokers
    (FANS)
PO Box 24052
Seattle,WA 98124
(206) 282-5565
(206) 932-7011

WEST VIRGINIA

Kathi K. Elkins
Federation of Active Non-
    smokers
PO Box 3980
Charleston, WV 25339
(304) 342-6600

WISCONSIN

Richard D. Dreiser
Southern Wisconsin GASP
1342 Pleasant Street
Lake Geneva, WI 53147

WYOMING

Linda Koldenhoven
Wyoming GASP
2672 Jefferson
Laramie, WY 82070
(307) 745-9338

APPENDIX B

Sample Nonsmokers' Rights Ordinances: San Diego and San Francisco, California

This appendix includes two model nonsmokers' rights laws. They are all strong, and address the most important areas where smokers and nonsmokers come in contact. Perhaps most important, they all place the right to breathe smokefree air above the privilege to smoke.

SAN DIEGO

ORDINANCE NO. 0-15865 (New Series), (0-83-63 Revised), Adopted on *Dec. 6, 1982*.

AN ORDINANCE AMENDING CHAPTER IV, ARTICLE 5, DIVISION 1 OF THE *SAN DIEGO MUNICIPAL CODE* BY AMENDING SECTIONS 45.0101, 45.0102, 45.0103, 45.0104, 45.0105, 45.0107 AND 45.0108 RELATING TO REGULATION OF SMOKING IN PUBLIC PLACES AND PLACES OF EMPLOYMENT.

BE IT ORDAINED, by the Council of the City of San Diego, as follows:

Section 1. That Chapter IV, Article 5, Division 1 of the San Diego Municipal Code be and it is hereby amended by amending Sections 45.0101, 45.0102, 45.0103, 45.0104, 45.0105, 45.0107 and 45.0108 to read as follows:

SEC. 45.0101—Purpose of Article

Because smoking of tobacco, or any other weed or plant, is a positive danger to health and a material annoyance, inconvenience, discomfort, and a health hazard to those who are present in confined spaces, and in order to serve public health, safety, and welfare, the declared purpose of this Article is to prohibit the smoking of tobacco, or any weed or plant, in public places and places of employment except in designated smoking areas.

SEC. 45.0102—Definitions

"Smoke" or "smoking" as defined in this Article means and includes the carrying of a lighted pipe, or lighted cigar, or lighted cigarette of any kind, or the lighting of a pipe, cigar, or cigarette of any kind.

"Public place" means any enclosed area to which the public is invited or in which the public is permitted, including, but not limited to, retail stores, retail service establishments, retail food production and marketing establishments, restaurants, theatres, waiting rooms, reception areas, educational facilities, health facilities, and public transportation facilities. A private residence is not a "public place."

"Place of employment" means any enclosed area under the control of a public or private employer which employees normally frequent during the course of employment, including, but not limited to, work areas, employee lounges, conference rooms, and employee cafeterias. A private residence is not a "place of employment."

SEC. 45.0103—Prohibitions

No person shall smoke in a public place or place of employment except in designated smoking areas.

SEC. 45.0104—Designation of Smoking Areas

(a) Smoking areas may be designated in public places and places of employment by proprietors or other persons in charge except in retail stores, retail service establishments, food markets, public conveyances, theaters, auditoriums, public assembly rooms, meeting rooms, rest rooms, elevators, pharmacies, libraries, museums or galleries which are open to the public, or any other place where smoking is prohibited by the Fire Marshal or by other law, ordinance or regulation. Where smoking areas are designated, existing physical barriers and ventilation systems shall be used to minimize the toxic effect of smoke in adjacent nonsmoking areas. It shall be the responsibility of employers to provide smokefree areas for nonsmokers within existing facilities to the maximum extent possible but employers are not required to incur any expense to make structural or other physical modifications in providing these areas. An employer who in good faith develops and promulgates a policy regarding smoking and nonsmoking in the workplace shall be deemed to be in compliance with this section provided that a policy which designates an entire workplace as a smoking area shall not be deemed a good-faith policy.

Restaurants covered by the provisions of this Article shall designate an adequate amount of seating capacity to sufficiently meet the demands and shall inform all patrons that a no-smoking section is provided. No public place other than the ones enumerated in Section 45.0107 shall be designated as a smoking area in its entirety.

(b) Notwithstanding any other provision of this Article, any facility or area may be designated in its entirety as a no-smoking area by the owner or manager thereof.

SEC. 45.0105—Posting of Signs

Signs which designate smoking or no-smoking areas established by this Article shall be clearly, sufficiently, and conspicuously posted in every room, building, or other place so covered by this Article. No-smoking signs shall be specifically placed in retail food production and marketing establishments, including grocery stores and supermarkets open to the public, so that they are clearly visible to persons upon entering the store, clearly visible to persons in checkout lines, and clearly visible to persons at meat and produce counters. The manner of such posting including the wording, size, color, design, and place of posting whether on the walls, doors, tables, counters, stands, or elsewhere shall be at the discretion of the owner, operator, manager, or other person having control of such room, building, or other place so long as clarity, sufficiency, and conspicuousness are apparent in communicating the intent of this Article.

SEC. 45.0106—Governmental Agency Cooperation

The City Manager shall annually request such governmental and educational agencies involved with their specific business within the City of San Diego to establish local operating procedures to cooperate and comply with this ordinance. In Federal, State, County, and special school districts within the City of San Diego, the City Manager shall urge enforcement of their existing no-smoking prohibitions and request cooperation with this ordinance.

SEC. 45.0107—Exceptions

(a) No-smoking areas are not required in individual private offices, hotel and motel meeting and assembly rooms rented to guests, areas and rooms while in use for private social functions, private hospital rooms, psychiatric facilities, jails, bars, stores that deal exclusively in tobacco products and accessories, and restaurants or eating establishments with a seating capacity of less than 20 persons.

(b) Restaurants or eating establishments with a seating capacity of less than 20 persons shall have the option of designating a no-smoking section or allowing or prohibiting smoking throughout the establishment.

(c) Any owner or manager of a business or other establishment subject to this Article may apply to the City Council for an exemption or modification of the provisions of this Article due to unique or unusual circumstances or conditions.

SEC. 45.0108—Enforcement and Appeal

(a) The City Manager shall be responsible for compliance with this Article when facilities which are owned, operated, or leased by the

City of San Diego are involved. The City Manager shall provide business license applicants with copies of this Article.

(b) The owner, operator or manager of any facility, business or agency shall post or cause to be posted all "No Smoking" signs required by this Article. Owners, operators, managers, or employees of same shall be required to orally inform persons violating this Article of the provisions thereof. The duty to inform such violator shall arise when such owner, operator, manager, or employee of same becomes aware of such violation.

(c) It shall be the responsibility of employers to disseminate information concerning the provisions of this Article to employees.

(d) The provisions of this Article pertaining to places of employment shall not apply until July 1, 1984.

SEC. 45.0109—Violations and Penalties

Any person who violates any provision of this article by smoking in a posted "No Smoking" area, or by failing to post or cause to be posted a "No Smoking" sign required by this article, or by a knowing failure to inform any person who violates the provision of this article, when such duty to inform arises as set forth in Section 45.0108, subsection (b) above, is guilty of an infraction and, upon conviction thereof, shall be punished by a fine of not less than ten dollars ($10) nor more than one hundred dollars ($100).

SEC. 45.0110—Education for No-Smoking Program

The City Manager, through the office of Citizens Assistance and Information, shall engage in a continuing program to inform and clarify the purposes of this article to citizens affected by it, and to guide owners, operators, and managers in their compliance.

The City shall leave the responsibility of conducting a public education campaign, regarding the health-degrading aspects of smoking, to other governmental and health agencies equipped with the needed expertise to conduct such campaigns.

SEC. 45.0111—Severability

If any provision, clause, sentence, or paragraph of this article or the application thereof to any person or circumstances shall be held invalid, such invalidity shall not affect the other provisions or application of the provisions of this article which can be given effect without the invalid provision or application, and to this end the provisions of this article are hereby declared to be severable.

Section 2. This ordinance shall take effect and be in force on the thirtieth day from and after its passage.

APPROVED: John W. Witt, City Attorney

By: _____

Stuart H. Swett
Chief Deputy City Attorney

SHS:rc:605
10/21/81 REV.11/15/82
Or.Dept:PS&S

SAN FRANCISCO

FILE NO. 158-82, ORDINANCE NO. 298-83 (Health Regulations).
AMENDING PART II, CHAPTER V, OF THE SAN FRANCISCO MUNICIPAL CODE (HEALTH CODE) BY ADDING ARTICLE 19 THERETO, REGULATING SMOKING IN THE OFFICE WORK-PLACE. NOTE: THE ENTIRE ARTICLE IS NEW.

Be it ordained by the People of the City and County of San Francisco:

Section 1. Part II, Chapter V, of the San Francisco Municipal Code (Health Code) is hereby amended by adding Article 19 thereto, reading as follows:

ARTICLE 19—Smoking Pollution Control

Sec. 1000—Title
Sec. 1001—Purpose

Sec. 1000—Title

This Article shall be known as the Smoking Pollution Control Ordinance.

Sec. 1001—Purpose

Because the smoking of tobacco or any other weed or plant is a danger to health and is a cause of material annoyance and discomfort to those who are present in confined places, the Board of Supervisors hereby declares that the purposes of this article are (1) to protect the public health and welfare by regulating smoking in the office workplace and (2) to minimize the toxic effects of smoking in the office workplace by requiring an employer to adopt a policy that will accommodate, insofar as possible, the preferences of nonsmokers and smokers and, if a satisfactory accommodation cannot be reached, to prohibit smoking in the office workplace.

This ordinance is not intended to create any right to smoke or to impair or alter an employer's prerogative to prohibit smoking in the workplace. Rather, if an employer allows employees to smoke in the workplace, then this ordinance requires (1) that the employer make accommodations for the preferences of both nonsmoking and smoking employees, and (2) if a satisfactory accommodation to all affected nonsmoking employees cannot be reached, that the employer prohibit smoking in the office workplace.

Sec. 1002—Definitions

For the purposes of this Article:
(1) "City" means the City and County of San Francisco;

(2) "Board of Supervisors" means the Board of Supervisors of the City and County of San Francisco;

(3) "Person" means any individual person, firm, partnership, association, corporation, company, organization, legal entity of any kind;

(4) "Employer" means any person who employs the service of an individual person;

(5) "Employee" means any person who is employed by any employer in consideration for direct or indirect monetary wage or profit;

(6) "Office Workplace" means any enclosed area of a structure or portion thereof intended for occupancy by business entities which will provide primarily clerical, professional, or business services of the business entity, or which will provide primarily clerical, professional, or business services to other business entities or to the public, at that location. Office workplace includes, but is not limited to, office spaces in office buildings, medical office waiting rooms, libraries, museums, hospitals, and nursing homes;

(7) "Smoking" or "to smoke" means and includes inhaling, exhaling, burning, or carrying any lighted smoking equipment for tobacco or any other weed or plant; and

(8) "Enclosed" means closed in by a roof and four walls with appropriate openings for ingress and egress and is not intended to mean areas commonly described as public lobbies.

Sec. 1003—Regulation of Smoking in the Office Workplace

(1) Each employer who operates an office or offices in the city shall within three (3) months of adoption of this ordinance, adopt, implement, and maintain a written Smoking Policy which shall contain, at a minimum, the following provisions and requirements:

(a) Any nonsmoking employee may object to his or her employer about smoke in his or her workplace. Using already available means of ventilation or separation or partition of office space, the employer shall attempt to reach a reasonable accommodation, insofar as possible, between the preferences of nonsmoking and smoking employees. However, an employer is not required by this ordinance to make any expenditures of structural changes to accommodate the preferences of nonsmoking or smoking employees.

(b) If an accommodation which is satisfactory to all affected nonsmoking employees cannot be reached in any given office workplace, the preferences of nonsmoking employees shall prevail and the employer shall prohibit smoking in that office workplace. Where the employer prohibits smoking in an office workplace, the area in which smoking is prohibited shall be clearly marked with signs.

(2) The Smoking Policy shall be announced within three (3) weeks of adoption to all employees working in office workplaces in the city and posted conspicuously in all workplaces under the employer's jurisdiction.

Sec. 1004—Where Smoking Not Regulated

This Article is not intended to regulate smoking in the following places and under the following conditions within the city:

(1) A private home which may serve as an office workplace;

(2) Any property owned or leased by state or federal governmental entities;

(3) Any office space leased or rented by a sole independent contractor;

(4) A private enclosed office workplace occupied exclusively by smokers, even though such an office workplace may be visited by nonsmokers, excepting places in which smoking is prohibited by the fire marshal or by other law, ordinance, or regulation; and:

Sec. 1005—Penalties and Enforcement

(1) The Director of Public Health shall enforce Section 1003 hereof against violations by either of the following actions:

(a) Serving notice requiring the correction of any violation of this Article;

(b) Calling upon the City Attorney to maintain an action for injunction to enforce the provisions of this Article, to cause the correction of any such violation, and for assessment and recovery of a civil penalty for such violation;

(2) Any employer who violates Section 1003 hereof may be liable for a civil penalty, not to exceed $500, which penalty shall be assessed and recovered in a civil action brought in the name of the People of the City and County of San Francisco in any court of competent jurisdiction. Each day such violation is committed or permitted to continue shall constitute a separate offense and shall be punishable as such. Any penalty assessed and recovered in an action brought pursuant to this paragraph shall be paid to the Treasurer of the City and County of San Francisco.

(3) In undertaking the enforcement of this ordinance, the City and County of San Francisco is assuming an undertaking only to promote the general welfare. It is not assuming, nor is it imposing on its officers and employees, an obligation for breach of which it is liable in money damages to any party of the state, that such breach proximately caused injury.

APPROVED AS TO FORM:
GEORGE AGHOST, City Attorney

By: _____
      Deputy City Attorney
1538C

Glossary of Tobacco Industry Euphemisms

They say you can't tell the players without a scorecard. Well, the same is true about the language used by the tobacco companies—smokespeak. It's a crazy universe where people who promote a product that causes people to die, call people who want to curtail smoking, "fanatics." In the tobacco world, the industry says it is trying to protect the "rights" of people whose numbers decline by over 350,000 a year because of cigarettes. Below is a brief compendium of cigarette company vocabulary and what each word or phrase really means:

Tobacco Vocabulary	*Meaning*
adult choice (as in the choice to smoke)	physical addiction
annoyance (as in tobacco smoke)	dangerous (as in tobacco smoke)
a political factor being inserted into the science	The Surgeon General's report is damaging to the tobacco industry

Tobacco Vocabulary	*Meaning*
biological change	something, that because nobody can see it, apparently doesn't happen—but does
claimed risks (as in risks claimed to be associated with smoking)	the warnings that appear on the cigarette packages, in medical journals, and from the Surgeon General, which can't be acknowledged because doing so would pave the way to successful product-liability suits against the cigarette companies
common courtesy	letting smokers smoke wherever they want
environmental tobacco smoke	disease-producing smoke
excessive government regulations	laws that protect the health of non-smokers, but that hurt the tobacco companies
free choice	overwhelming smokers with over $2 billion a year in advertising
habit	physical addiction
just epidemiological	the truth
just statistics	the truth
low nicotine	low poison
low tar	low poison
marketplace	preserving the status quo as long as the status quo allows smoking everywhere
no dose-response relationship	because scientists don't know everything about smoking, they don't know anything

Tobacco Vocabulary	Meaning
scientific conferences (also international conferences)	open meetings where pro-tobacco papers are presented (frequently sponsored by the Tobacco Institute)
scientific integrity	the tobacco point of view
smokers' rights	cigarette companies' need to make profits
sampling	giving teenagers free cigarettes so that they can become addicted

Index